BARRY J. SESSLE is in the Division of Biological Sciences at the Faculty of Dentistry, University of Toronto.
ALAN G. HANNAM is in the Department of Oral Biology at the Faculty of Dentistry, University of British Columbia.

Mastication and swallowing are functions common to most forms of animal life, yet there exists much uncertainty as to their biological basis, and a diversity of opinion on the treatment of disorders of the masticatory and deglutitory apparatus. During the last fifteen years there has been a considerable increase in research into clinical aspects related to these two vital functions, and also into their underlying biological, and especially neurophysiological, mechanisms.

This volume presents the edited proceedings of a symposium held in 1974 in Vancouver, British Columbia, attended by scientists from several countries who are actively involved in such research.

In addition to a broad, up-to-date coverage of its subject, *Mastication and Swallowing* stresses conceptual aspects and suggests lines of future clinical and basic research.

Mastication and Swallowing

Biological and clinical correlates

edited by
BARRY J. SESSLE
ALAN G. HANNAM

University of Toronto Press
TORONTO AND BUFFALO

© University of Toronto Press 1976
Toronto and Buffalo
Printed in Canada
Reprinted in 2018

Library of Congress Cataloging in Publication Data
Main entry under title:

Mastication and swallowing.

'Based on the proceedings of a symposium held on 5-8 August 1974 at the University
of British Columbia, Vancouver, Canada.'
Includes bibliographies and index.
1. Mastication – Congresses. 2. Deglutition – Congresses. I. Sessle, Barry J., 1941-
II. Hannam, Alan G., 1939-   [DNLM: 1. Mastication – Congresses. 2. Deglutition –
Congresses. WI102 M423 1974]
QP146.M37   612'.31   75-38957
ISBN 0-8020-2207-3
ISBN 978-1-4875-7280-8 (paper)

Contributors

P.G. DELLOW Health Sciences Centre, University of Western Ontario, London, Ont. N6A 3K7, Canada

RONALD DUBNER Neurobiology and Anesthesiology Branch, National Institutes of Health, Bethesda, Md. 20014, USA

STEPHEN GOBEL Neurobiology and Anesthesiology Branch, National Institutes of Health, Bethesda, Md. 20014, USA

L.J. GOLDBERG School of Dentistry, The Center for the Health Sciences, University of California, Los Angeles, Calif. 90024, USA

L.F. GREENWOOD Faculty of Dentistry, University of Toronto, 124 Edward St, Toronto, Ont. M5G 1G6, Canada

ALAN G. HANNAM Faculty of Dentistry, University of British Columbia, Vancouver, BC V6T 1W5, Canada

Y. KAWAMURA Department of Oral Physiology, Dental School, Osaka University, Kitaku, Osaka, Japan

KISOU KUBOTA Department of Neurophysiology, Primate Research Institute, Kyoto University, Inuyama, Aichi, 484, Japan

J.P. LUND Faculté de Médecine dentaire et Centre de Recherches en Science Neurologique, Université de Montréal, Case postale 6208, Montréal, PQ H3C 3T8, Canada

A.A. LOWE Faculty of Dentistry, University of Toronto, 124 Edward St, Toronto, Ont. M5G 1G6, Canada

BRUCE MATTHEWS Department of Physiology, Medical School, University Walk, Bristol BS8 1TD, England

E. MØLLER Department of Electromyography, Royal Dental College, Jagtvej 160, Copenhagen DK2100, Denmark

R.H. ROYDHOUSE Department of Restorative Dentistry, Faculty of Dentistry, University of British Columbia, Vancouver, BC V6T 1W5, Canada

BARRY J. SESSLE Faculty of Dentistry, University of Toronto, 124 Edward St, Toronto, Ont. M5G 1G6, Canada

A.T. STOREY Faculty of Dentistry, University of Toronto, 124 Edward St, Toronto, Ont. M5G 1G6, Canada

TADAAKI SUMI Department of Physiology, Fujita-Gakuen University, School of Medicine, Toyoake, Nagoya, Japan 470-11

N.R. THOMAS Faculty of Dentistry, University of Alberta, Edmonton, Alta. T6G 2H7, Canada

Contents

SECTION FOUR
Mastication and swallowing: patterning and controls of muscle activity

SECTION FIVE
Workshop group reports

Preface

This book is based on the proceedings of a symposium held on 5–8 August 1974 at the University of British Columbia, Vancouver, Canada. The symposium brought together an international group of scientists actively involved in research into clinical and biological aspects of mastication and swallowing. It thus presented a rare opportunity for a highly respected group of researchers in these fields to interact and thereby consolidate and clarify present concepts of the two processes.

Mastication and swallowing provide most interesting systems from both clinical and biological viewpoints. The maintenance of a high level of performance of these basic functions is the goal of many clinical areas in dentistry and allied fields. Both functions are also intriguing to the biologist since they represent two rather different patterns or paradigms of behaviour. Mastication is manifested as a cyclical, learned pattern that may be susceptible to sensory feedback and modification, whereas swallowing has been shown to be a triggered, all-or-none, and apparently unlearned, activity that is largely independent of such feedback. Both functions, moreover, are fundamental yet highly complicated and coordinated functions of man and lower animals. The complexity of these functions and the variety of factors (e.g. pain, hunger, stress, emotion) that can influence their expression have resulted in much uncertainty about their underlying biological mechanisms and about the treatment of disorders of the masticatory and deglutitory apparatus.

Nevertheless, over the last fifteen years, there has been a marked increase in interest and study of clinical aspects of chewing and swallowing and their underlying biological mechanisms. However, there have been very few attempts to correlate this recent knowledge, and there seems to be no book solely devoted to this subject which has such clinical and biological relevance. Thus the published proceedings of this symposium, in providing a definitive up-to-date and wide coverage of mastication and swallowing, should be of immeasurable value and interest to physiologists, clinicians, and specialists in dentistry and allied fields, students in these areas, and dental researchers and teachers.

By way of formal papers, discussions, and workshops, the participants in the symposium reviewed and presented both defined and conceptual aspects of the neuromuscular mechanisms involved in mastication and swallowing. These mechanisms were related, where possible, to clinical manifestations of normal and altered function. The participants also pointed out profitable areas and lines of future clinical and basic research in these fields. The outcome of these deliberations and ideas are presented here.

The book is divided into five sections. The first four deal with various facets of mastication and swallowing, ranging from their general aspects (Section One) to specific considerations of underlying mechanisms (Section Two) and factors such as pain which can influence mastication, swallowing, and associated oral-facial motility patterns (Sections Three and Four). Each paper is based on review material and recent research results and is followed by an edited general discussion that involved all participants. A chairman's summary of the main points of the session concludes each section. The last section deals with the deliberations of three workshop groups which addressed themselves to three specific questions with both clinical and biological overtones. The groups attempted to answer the questions using the information gained from the preceding four sessions, plus additional information obtained from the clinical and basic science literature. The reports in this book represent the highlights of their deliberations and of the subsequent general discussion that followed the presentation of each workshop group's findings by its chairman. All presentations in each section have a separate bibliography which, together with the index at the back of the book, makes this volume suitable for ready reference.

At the last moment, illness forced the withdrawal from the meeting of Drs E. Møller, Royal Dental College, Copenhagen, and D.J. Kenny, Faculty of Dentistry, University of Toronto. Fortunately Dr Møller's paper was presented for him, and Dr Møller contributed to the ensuing discussion in writing.

The symposium was held with the support of the Medical Research Council of Canada and the Ministry of Health of the Province of British Columbia. The Ministry also subsidized publication of this book, and we gratefully acknowledge the generous support of both agencies. The participants are grateful to the University of British Columbia for its hospitality, and thanks are especially due to Drs R.H. Roydhouse and P.G. Dellow, and the Department of Oral Biology, University of British Columbia, for help in local arrangements for the symposium. We are grateful to Ms B. Holmwood for her editorial assistance, to Ms D. Tsang who handled correspondence and typing, and Ms L. Ouram and Ms G. Stevenson and staff of the University of Toronto Press for their assistance in the publication.

Toronto, March 1975   B.J.S.
                                                             A.G.H.

SECTION ONE

Mastication and swallowing in perspective

Chairman's Introduction

N.R. THOMAS

How the central nervous system produces coordinated motor output and appropriate inhibition of competing activities has been of major concern to physiologists. Because of the functional and anatomical complexities of cranial organization, the continuous alternation of jaw elevators and depressors as in mastication or the sequential contraction of bucco-pharyngo-oesophageal musculature as in deglutition provide an even more fascinating study for those interested in integrative physiology. This first session aims to provide an overall view of these processes in the general physiological context.

Until recently control theories have been based on linked reflexes dependent upon sensory feedback (Sherrington, 1917). It has however been demonstrated by various means (e.g. Doty, Richmond, and Storey, 1967; Dellow and Lund, 1971) that the central nervous system, once triggered, sends patterned instructions specific for mastication and deglutition to the appropriate muscles at the appropriate level of excitation/inhibition and in proper temporal relationship and in the absence of phase-to-phase afferent feedback from the periphery. Nevertheless, it is also recognized that under physiological conditions, peripheral feedback operates to modulate the swallow or chew pattern as clinically illustrated by the lip incompetent 'tongue-thrust swallow' or the 'bite of accommodation' in cases of malocclusion.

The neurones responsible for the coordination of mastication have been placed in a region of reticular formation adjacent to the rostral end of the mesencephalic nucleus of the trigeminal nerve (Woods, 1964; Parker and Feldman, 1967; Thomas, 1969) and for swallowing to bilateral areas of the reticular formation rostro-dorsally to the inferior olives (Doty et al., 1967). These neurones of the so-called chewing and swallowing 'centres' form functional neurone groups interconnected in such a manner as to produce automatically, when effectively excited, inhibitory and excitatory sequences in appropriate motoneurones.

Triggering of these 'centres' requires a 'decision' by the central nervous system that certain criteria have been met. Convergence of appropriate input on a single cell may initiate the single impulse that releases the complex patterns. Another explanation is that a network of interacting neurones has a threshold different from that for any constituent cell. The excitability of this network as a whole must reach a definite level before it becomes active. It is also known that the 'centres' contain subcentres, and partial destruction of the centre produces a number of fractionations of activity (Doty, 1968). It is possible that such fractions or subsynergies are accessible as important elements of other patterned responses (e.g. speech). Since a variety of reflexes can be elicited utilizing this neurone pool, the afferent gate for swallowing and mastication must be so organized as to accept only those stimulus patterns having a certain spatio-temporal code. In this respect it is well established that stimulation of specific regions of the cortex (orbital, prefrontal lobes, etc.), striatum (including amygdala and subthalamic nuclei, etc.), thalamus, and brain stem reticular formation evokes chewing and swallowing after a lengthy latent period.

When the 'Hunger-Centre' or lateral hypothalamic nucleus, with its rich connections to the brain above and brain stem regions, is stimulated, similar responses of chewing and swallowing occur. In view of the functional relationship of the reticular formation to all these regions and particularly to the swallowing and masticatory 'centres,' it is not surprising that the administration of agents mimicking or inhibitory to the endogenous neurotransmitters of the reticular activating system should stimulate or inhibit chewing and swallowing respectively. Indeed, evidence has been accumulated that the brain aminergic transmitters involved are directly influenced by dietary intake and hence may function as important transducers in the hunger response.

Obviously swallowing must interact with respiration, but there is considerable evidence that other activities interact with swallowing and mastication such as cardiomotor, vasomotor, locomotion, and pain transmission processes (Doty, 1968; Lund and Dellow, 1971). The state of maturity of the central nervous system dictates the relative priority of one activity over another. Thus it is of great interest to neurophysiologists to elucidate the mechanisms by which this is achieved. We have only just begun to investigate the effects of endogenous feedback loops in the initiation and control of coordinated movements generally and I suspect that researches into swallowing and mastication control will be very profitable in this regard, particularly as Renshaw loops have not been demonstrated for cranial nerves involved in these activities.

REFERENCES

Dellow, P.G., and Lund, J.P. 1971. Evidence for central timing of rhythmical mastication. *J. Physiol. (Lond.)* 215: 1-13

Doty, R.W. 1968. Neural organisation of deglutition. In C.F. Code (ed.), *Handbook of Physiology.* Vol. IV, Sect. 6. Washington: Physiol. Soc.

Doty, R.W., Richmond, W.H., and Storey, A.T. 1967. Effect of medullary lesions on co-ordination of deglutition. *Exp. Neurol.* 17: 91-106

Lund, J.P., and Dellow, P.G. 1971. The influence of interactive stimuli on rhythmical masticatory movement in rabbits. *Archs oral Biol.* 16: 215-23

Parker, S.W., and Feldman, S.M. 1967. Effect of mesencephalic lesions on feeding behaviour in rats. *Exp. Neurol.* 17: 313-26

Sherrington, C.S. 1917. Reflexes elicitable in the cat from pinna, vibrissae and jaw. *J. Physiol. (Lond.)* 51: 404-31

Thomas, N.R. 1969. Reflex mastication and its central control in the decerebrate rat. *J. Canad. Dent. Assoc.* 35: 273

Woods, J.W. 1964. Behavior of chronic decerebrate rats. *J. Neurophysiol.* 27: 635-44

The general physiological background of chewing and swallowing

PETER G. DELLOW

There has been a long evolutionary progress of the eating apparatus up to that of man, although man cannot be said to be particularly sophisticated in his ability to eat. The progress comes through the other functions to which man puts the special apparatus. Nevertheless he must ingest, as any animal, to live: and sucking, drinking, chewing, and swallowing are important human behaviours. The placement of dietary likes in a mouth is a basic phenomenon common to man and to many another animals. Ultimately these substances become the animal itself, whether it be a protozoan, a shark, or a human. Mastication is not essential to all forms of food intake or to a successful life: whales may filter-feed, and grow to an enormous size; some fish filter-feed also from their respiratory currents, and others swallow whole their lubricated prey; a frog may flick its tongue to catch an insect, and then swallow it unmasticated; and many reptiles are known for their ability to swallow intact animals. Deglutition is a much more general phenomenon. Man must always swallow, even though his need for mastication seems to be diminishing.

With the vitality, complexity, and necessary coordination of oropharyngeal functions in ingestion, it is not surprising that the physiological controls of ingestion are themselves complex. Indeed, our very knowledge of them is poor. The mechanisms of the basic drives to eat and drink are even more elusive topics than the motor acts themselves. Millennia of evolutionary development have dictated the instinctual, the automatic, and the sentient ingestive acts of man. Thus it is interesting to reflect upon control structures which have developed out of a close biological relationship to the mouth or portal of entry of food and water. A brain is such a structure; a case can be made for the development of this as a correlate of food ingestion. And the liaison between mouth and brain is figuratively cemented by the outgrowths of the anterior and posterior hypophysis. These, with the attendant hypothalamus, are key control organs – influencing all tissues and the tissue relationships with essential ingested materials. Other chemocontrollers develop from oropharyngeal structures, illustrating a theoretical need to commence, from the local level, the management or balance of materials that pass through the mouth. Thyroid, parathyroid, tonsillar, ultimobranchial, thymic, and carotid and aortic glomus tissues evolve and assist in the management of the internal environment. There are also evidences for endocrine roles of the salivary glands and for chemical influences of saliva at more distant sites in the digestive tract.

Although a close physical oropharyngeal association of many of the controllers would appear to be phylogenetic, the representative liaison with the brain is large and obvious. This can be found in the innervation density, several vegetative centres, the large somatotopy within sensorimotor areas, related special senses, speech control, elements of the psyche, and in the multiple limbic zones related to consummatory behaviour. The central nervous relation also allows an integration of orofacial and oropharyngeal function with the functions of other parts and organs, and with behaviours other than the consummatory.

Oral and pharyngeal motor activity commences in the foetus, as exhibited by the drinking of amniotic fluid, sucking movements, and the occasional presentation of a thumb between the lips. One might suspect that facial contortions also occur. Amniotic fluid differs in composition from foetal tissue fluid and undoubtedly saliva, so a chemical stimulus may exist through its sapidity. Certainly, more is swallowed if it is sweetened with glucose. The noted performances can be regarded as training for the crucial act of sucking in the post-natal period. Indeed, the daily volume of amniotic fluid swallowed shortly before birth matches that of mother's milk ingested just after birth. One thus wonders if there might not be some learning involved in, at least, the act of sucking, paralleling intrauterine developments in muscles, nerves, and the central nervous system. Certainly, by the time of viable birth the act is instinctual and automatic, apparently reflexogenic, and coupled to the distinctly reflex act of deglutition. The postulate can be extended further in implicating learning in the act of mastication, with a degree of automaticity subsequently being supplanted on the learnt pattern and perhaps utilizing the rhythm-controller of sucking as a base. Extra-uterine aging, the eruption of teeth, environmental manipulations by the mouth, sapid experiences, and the maternal introductions of different foods assist in the development of a learnt behaviour of mastication. A security of motor engrams in an experienced and more mature brain allows the automaticity. The latter never supersedes the volitional element, and certainly it is not similar to the synergy of deglutition whose automaticity is reflexogenic and irrefutable as it is triggered from the oropharyngeal, pharyngeal, and laryngeal zones.

Activities which, to all intents and purposes, are visceral but which are undertaken by striped musculature apparently deserve special brain stem controls. Thus we find reticular neuronal assemblies concerned with the behaviours of rhythmical sucking and lapping, deglutition, vomiting, and respiration. The former acts are very much linked to smooth muscle performances in the gut; and they, along with glandular activity, assist the more acceptable visceration that is digestion and absorption. The rhythm of walking is also apparently in-built in the central nervous system. Likewise tail-wagging, which may show an exhibited rate paralleling that of the pleasant behaviour of sucking milk from the cud. These tail, limb, thoracic cage, jaw, and tongue rhythms involve conjoint or reciprocal effects extending across the midline of the nervous system; and, although influenced by suprasegmental structures, they are not dependent upon higher nervous function. Anencephalic neonates do undertake sucking and certain other fundamental or visceral behaviours concerned with the acquisition of nutrients. Reflex salivary activity occurs along with the activity in the striped musculature as the food is ingested; control of this secretion is also through brain stem regulatory centres.

The overall actions of the upper end of the gastrointestinal tract are thus quite similar to those further down where there is less of a dependence upon central nervous control. There is a nice parade of activities for food intake: given a certain degree of development, there is the voluntary placement of food in the mouth, its mastication as necessary (this being voluntary and/or rhythmically automatic), the automatic synergy of cranio-cervical musculature in swallowing once reflexly triggered, and the continuance of the swallowing performance in the involuntary muscle beyond the mid-oesophagus. Transgression further into and through the gut continues by the in-built activities of its smooth muscle, with some overlay control through intrinsic and extrinsic autonomic nerves. Special central nervous centres are not now necessary, either for the motor activities of different segments of the gut or for the integrated responses of the glands. The vagus nerve, nevertheless, does have some allegiance to the brain stem visceral centres and it does also have supervisory control effects over a large amount of the gut. Sympathetic and parasympathetic centres, also with wide influences, can be found in the hypothalamus. A great dependence on chemical signals is apparent in the true gut. At the oral end it is much less if one evades the phylogenetic concept previously discussed; it is, nevertheless, manifest in the taste sense. Some chemical control through oral absorption is a possibility, and there may be salivary endocrine principles with metabolic functions. Within the hypothalamus, chemical signals are important for the regulation of eating and drinking.

The respiratory centres in the brain stem have a recognized control over somatic musculature, and this can be both modulated by volition and stimulated by visceral signals. Sucking and lapping activity, and perhaps the substrate of automatic mastication, seem somewhat comparable. The stimulus for these is ordinarily the 'visceral' signal of acceptable food or fluid in the mouth, but internal signals may occasionally provoke jaw rhythms. These may be seen from time to time in the young in anticipation of food, and in the elderly, having a basis in a possible degenerative breakdown of supraseg-mental inhibitory mechanisms. The respiratory centres do interplay with the ingestive centres, perhaps best, but not exclusively, demonstrated by the cessation of respiration and by glottic closure during swallowing. Whilst these performances are reflexogenic or automatic, the voluntary control over respiration and the orofacial muscles reaches a superb and sophisticated maximum in man in his ability to talk. Subtending speech there is an element which is rhythmic, and it might be within our realm of postulation to consider this to be related to the sucking mechanism. Certainly there are elementary levels of the control of speech which are not neocortical, although a large proportion of the cerebral cortex is so specified. The rhythmic capabilities of groups of muscles might be evidenced in the mandibular tremor sometimes seen in stutterers. Be this as it may, the controllers of speech certainly output through musculature that is also active during ingestion.

While contemplating that a brain might have evolved because of a need to control the attainment of food, one can further speculate upon topics such as language giving vent through the ingestive apparatus, the fact that man thinks or romanticizes in terms of language, the role of the ingestive apparatus in the development of the psyche, the highly hedonistic value of chewing and swallowing, and concerning the exhibition of emotional expression through the face and mouth. Most of these topics cannot yet be discussed in terms of physiology, so perhaps one might best dwell upon more factual examples, some of which are illustrated in Figures 1-5. The numbers in parentheses in each figure legend indicate the appropriate references. These figures and their legends do no more than sample knowledge of the area; the intention is that they provide some background in physiology for the more particular works that follow.

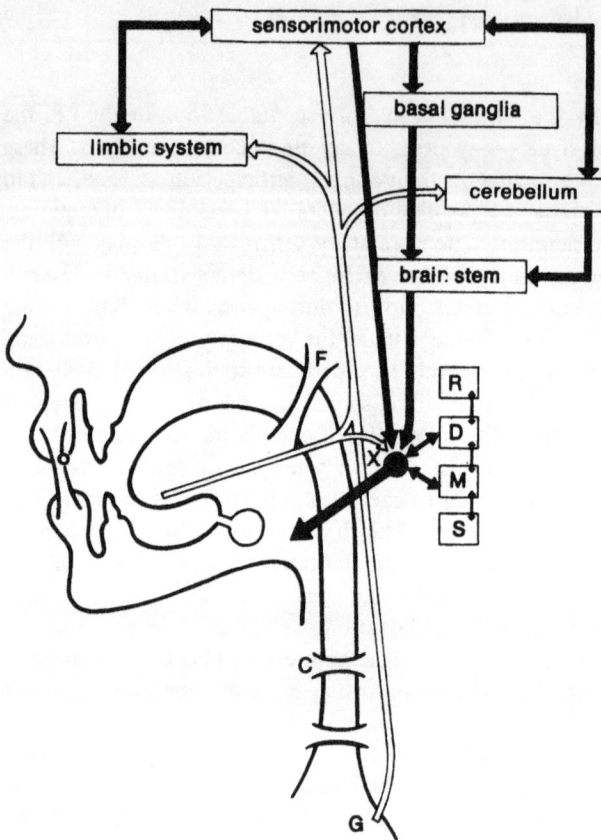

FIGURE 1 Hierarchical arrangement of the neural structures controlling movements in the ingestive apparatus. At the simplest level are the brain stem reflexes (X). These are allied to the neuronal assemblies associated with the basic controls of respiration (R), rhythmical sucking and mastication (M), deglutition (D), and salivation (S) (7, 10, 46, 51). The brain stem has general motor control sites in the reticular formation, pontine nuclei, cerebellar nuclei, red nucleus, and substantia nigra, while beyond this core, large neuronal pools in the cerebral cortex, limbic system, basal ganglia, motor thalamus, and cerebellum are involved in motor and behavioural control (6, 18, 27, 34, 41, 46). Sucking and swallowing movements sufficient for subservient sustenance can be adequately controlled through the interplay of brain stem mechanisms alone (6, 46). Ordinarily, automatic ingestive movements are keyed by the sensory inputs from appropriate material in the mouth and oropharynx, although non-nutritive sucking activity is normal in the neonate (47, 50). Sensory input channels influence all levels of motor control (40, 46, 53). There is some evidence that the reappearance of spontaneous rhythmical jaw movements in the aged is due to an imbalance of cholinergic and dopaminergic mechanisms in the caudate nucleus of the basal ganglia (25, 35, 49). In addition to such specific chemical paths in the brain, a release of hypothalamic neurohumors and substances released secondarily from the pituitary gland are relevant to the behavioural overlay of motor control (3, 9, 13, 31, 54). The neural outputs are to striated musculature except for those to salivary and mucous glands, blood vessels, and to the lower half of the oesophagus. The circumoral (O), faucial (F), and cricopharyngeal (C) muscles can be considered as sphincters of the digestive tract; and likewise the vocal cords can be a protective sphincter of the respiratory tree. The vocal cords act in concert with the oropharyngeal musculature during speech, and the motor control of this behaviour necessitates a large

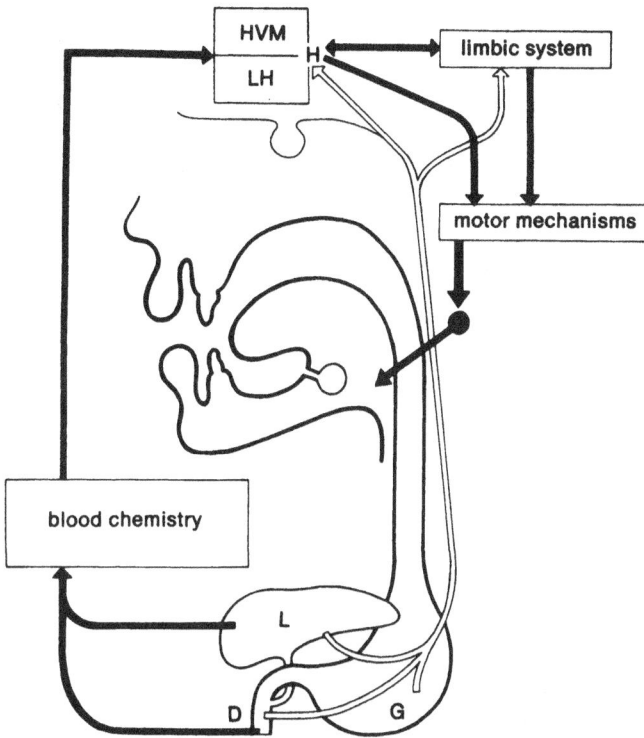

cortical involvement. The second major receptive organ of ingestion, the stomach (G), is naturally involved in control, particularly with pre-feeding inputs to the brain, post-ingestive inputs from distension, and conditioned responses (2, 42, 45). The tenth cranial nerve is its motor controller.

FIGURE 2 A general scheme for the behavioural control of food intake. Classical theory involves the hypothalamus (H) as a focal area which detects the need for sustenance or the need for cessation of ingestion through satiation (30, 55). Hypothalamic connections and neuroendocrine phenomena allow a wide span of control; and an influence over the frank sensory and motor mechanisms of the mouth and pharynx can be suggested (21, 30, 40, 41, 54). Duodenal (D), gastric (G), and hepatic (L) afferentations to the hypothalamus have been implicated as control signals; and specific hypothalamic cellular signalling from blood glucose, lipid, amino acid, cholecystokinin, osmolality, and temperature levels have also been postulated (1, 2, 4, 38, 44, 55). The strongest evidence is for glucoreceptors: indeed, the blood glucose level is said to rise within one minute of the ingestion of food, thus theoretically keying an early receptor mechanism for the impending cessation of eating (1, 33). A lowered blood glucose may be a correlate of hunger, and this is probably associated with an altered and increased afferentation from gastric movements and with an immediate metabolic 'inadequacy' in the musculature. A satiety centre in the ventromedial hypothalamus (HVM) and a feeding centre in the lateral hypothalamus (LH) form central sites in the control system, and these are linked to limbic and mesencephalic structures (1, 15, 17, 26, 30, 36, 37). The amygdala, septum, hippocampus, ventral tegmentum, and central gray are involved in the control of ingestive behaviour, and one must implicate all levels of motor control (6, 8, 21, 27, 30). There is a noradrenergic bias present in the control of feeding (3, 13, 31).

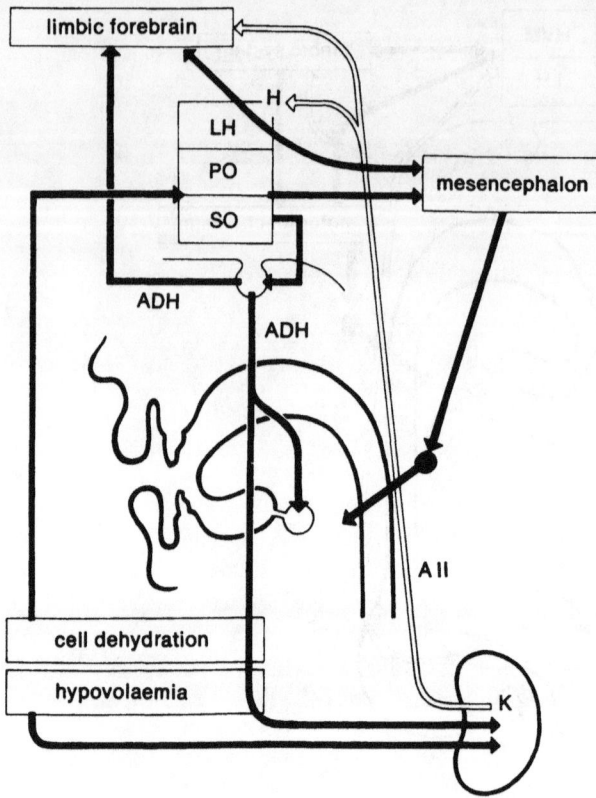

FIGURE 3 Mechanisms involved in the control of water intake. The need for repletion of body water appears to be detected by two sets of cells: the first responding to extracellular fluid volume, the second to intracellular dehydration. A fundamental avenue of the former is through the juxtaglomerular apparatus of the kidney (K) and the renin-angiotensin (AII) system. In addition to changes produced in sodium balance and fluid distribution within the body, renin and angiotensin appear also to have trigger effects in the brain motivational system for drinking (14). The hypothalamus (H), in particular the lateral hypothalamus (LH), is again a focal zone, and the amygdala, septum, ventral tegmentum, and cingulate cortex are also involved (14, 17, 30). Limbic and hypothalamic links to the mesencephalon exist, and these can be interpreted as an intercession with the more precise motor controls (30). There are pathways of association between the lateral hypothalamus and the hypothalamic preoptic (PO) and supraoptic (SO) nuclei; and it is these latter nuclei that have cells responsive to cellular dehydration (14). An additional drive to seek water is thereby instituted. At the same time, and by the same means, the supraoptic nucleus is stimulated to deliver and release antidiuretic hormone (ADH) from the neurohypophysis (9). Besides its effects on renal tubular mechanisms, there is also a possible influence of ADH on the limbic-hypothalamic mechanisms associated with the behavioural drive to seek replenishing water and on salivary gland secretion (14). Although a drying of the mouth and pharynx does form a part of the thirst mechanism, it is not now considered to be the principal source of the corrective drive (5, 14). Nevertheless, the osmotically sensitive hypothalamic cells do seem to receive lingual afferent activity induced by osmotic or gustatory changes in the mouth (11, 32). The central mechanisms of thirst appear to be dominantly cholinergic (15, 35).

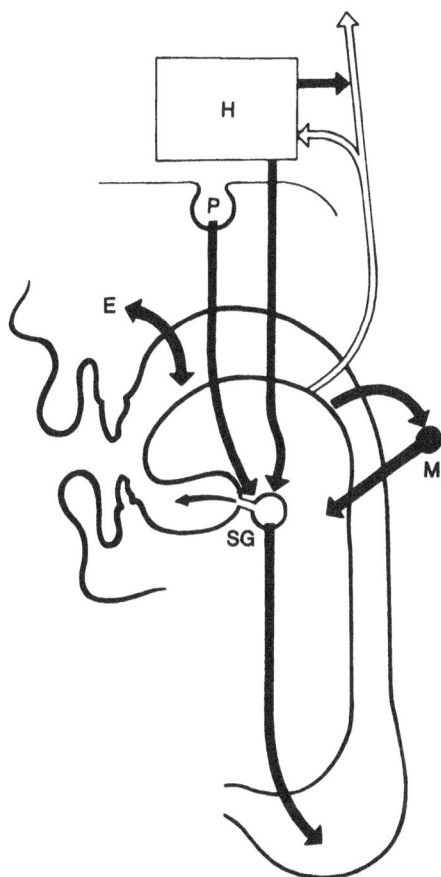

FIGURE 4 Some specific oral links that may have a role in the general physiological controls of ingestion. Drying of the mucous membrane is involved in the sensation of thirst, thus the salivary glands (SG) are brought into the general homeostatic scene (5). A central focus in the control of water and food intake is the hypothalamus (H), and there are also physiological influences of this basal brain area over the salivary glands (36, 37). One of these suggests a hypothalamic-parotid-tooth axis, with a humoral influence on fluid flow through dentine (20). Salivary glands are also susceptible to a conditioned response of feeding; and there is a possible hormonal influence from the salivary glands over gastric motor activity (28, 42). Fluid and molecular exchanges (E) do occur between the external and internal environments of the mouth, but it remains to be seen if these influence ingestive control (23, 29). The latter is certainly influenced by oral sensory activity; and there are orohypothalamic paths of a general and a gustatory nature (11, 21, 32, 40, 46, 47, 53). Hypothalamic activity has some control over oral sensory fields and in the orienting and response reactions to oral stimuli (24, 43). Oropharyngeal sensations interact with the ingestive controls of the hypothalamus, and they can also assist in triggering rhythmic jaw and tongue (M) movements (21, 26). Taste has a role in ingestion, especially in salt balance and in the energy gain through sweet substances (19, 52). Saliva is necessary for the taste sense, and this medium appears to receive some general endocrine modification; again, this allows a hypothalamic link through the pituitary gland (P). The latter, of course, has a profound influence on the maintenance of oral tissues (39).

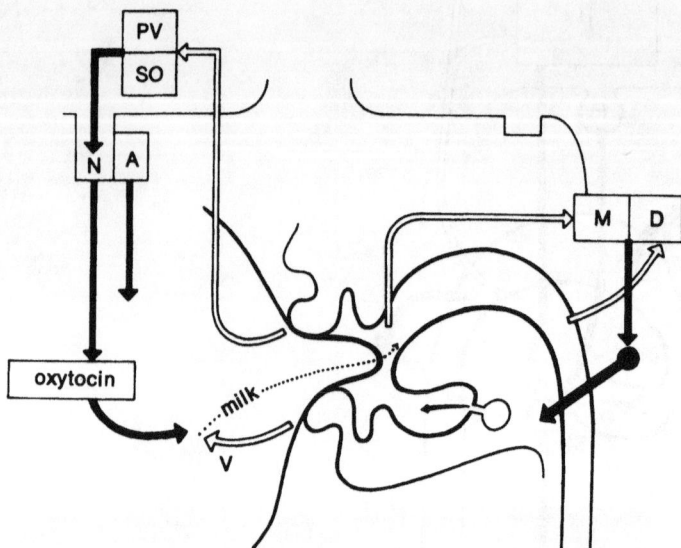

FIGURE 5 Elements in the conjoint response of mother and child in suckling. The automatic and rhythmical motor activity of the neonate, along with periodic swallowing, receives its integrated control from the hind brain (M, D), each act being triggered by appropriate stimuli of the anterior and of the posterior parts of the mouth (7, 8, 21, 47). All other things being equal, the cessation of an ingestive period of sucking is presumably through gastric distension and the post-absorptive chemical state influencing limbic and hypothalamic centres (38, 45). Tactile, muscular, and gustatory stimuli cause a reflex flow of saliva which assists in the labial seal on the nipple (12). The scene is also set for the development of the conditioned salivary response (42). The thrusting and closure of the infantile lips and gum pads upon the peri-areolar tissue is responsible for milk removal, but true physical sucking is a minimal factor (22). The main mechanism comes through the milk-ejection reflex of the mother; peri-areolar stimulation acts through the paraventricular (PV) and supraoptic (SO) nuclei of the hypothalamus to release oxytocin from the neurohypophysis (N), this in turn causing smooth muscle responses in the alveoli and lactiferous ducts (48). Milk production is assisted via prolactin of the adenohypophysis (A) while at the local level, the suckling act stimulates the release of vasodilator metabolites (V) which increase blood flow and favour milk production and release (16). The hypothalamic and renal controls of fluid balance are implicated in both individuals; the satiation of the infant at the expense of fluid loss and thirst in the mother.

REFERENCES

1 Anand, B.K., Dua, S., and Singh, B. 1961. Electrical activity of the hypothalamic 'feeding centres' under effect of changes in blood chemistry. *Electroenceph. clin. Neurophysiol.* 13: 54–9

2 Anand, B.K., and Pillai, R.V. 1967. Activity of single neurones in the hypo-thalamic feeding centres: effect of gastric distension. *J. Physiol. (Lond.)* 192: 63–77

3 Booth, D.A. 1968. Mechanism of action of norepinephrine in eliciting an eat-ing response on injections into the rat hypothalamus. *J. Pharmacol. exp. Ther.* 160: 336–48

4 Brobeck, J.R. 1960. Food and temperature. *Recent Progr. Hormone Res.* 16: 439–66

5 Cannon, W.B. 1918. The physiological basis of thirst. *Proc. Roy. Soc. (Lond.)* Ser. B. 90: 283–301

6 Dellow, P.G. 1969. Control mechanisms of mastication. *Ann. Aust. Coll. Dental Surg.* 2: 81–95

7 Dellow, P.G., and Lund, J.P. 1971. Evidence for central timing of rhythmical mastication. *J. Physiol. (Lond.)* 215: 1–13

8 Doty, R.W. 1968. Neural organization of deglutition. In C.F. Code (ed.), *Handbook of Physiology.* Vol. IV, Sect. 6. Washington: Am. Physiol. Soc.

9 Dreifuss, J.J., Kalnins, I., Kelly, J.S., and Ruf, K.B. 1971. Action potentials and release of neurohypophysial hormones in vitro. *J. Physiol. (Lond.)* 215: 805–17

10 Easton, T.A. 1972. On the normal use of reflexes. *Am. Sci.* 60: 591–9

11 Emmers, R. 1973. Interaction of neural systems which control body water. *Brain Res.* 49: 323–47

12 Epstein, A.N., Blass, E.M., Batshaw, M.L., and Parks, A.D. 1970. The vital role of saliva as a mechanical sealant for suckling in the rat. *Physiol. Behav.* 5: 1395–8

13 Evetts, K.D., Fitzsimons, J.T., and Setler, P.E. 1972. Eating caused by 6-hydroxydopamine-induced release of noradrenaline in the diencephalon of the rat. *J. Physiol. (Lond.)* 223: 35–47

14 Fitzsimons, J.T. 1972. Thirst. *Physiol. Rev.* 52: 468–561

15 Grossman, S.P. 1968. Hypothalamic and limbic influences on food intake. *Fed. Proc.* 27: 1349–60

16 Hanwell, A., and Linzell, J.L. 1973. The effects of engorgement with milk and of suckling on mammary blood flow in the rat. *J. Physiol. (Lond.)* 233: 111–25

17 Huang, Y.H., and Mogenson, G.J. 1972. Neural pathways mediating drinking and feeding in rats. *Exp. Neurol.* 37: 269–86

18 Kornhuber, H.H. 1974. Cerebral cortex, cerebellum, and basal ganglia: an introduction to their motor functions. In F.O. Schmitt and F.G. Worden (eds.), *The Neurosciences. Third Study Program.* Massachusetts: M.I.T. Press

19 LeMagnen, J. 1953. Activité de l'insuline sur la consommation spontanée des solutions sapides. *C.R. Soc. Biol.* 147: 1753-7

20 Leonora, J., and Steinman, R.R. 1968. Evidence suggesting the existence of a hypothalamic-parotid gland endocrine axis. *Endocrinol.* 83: 807-15

21 Lund, J.P., and Dellow, P.G. 1971. The influence of interactive stimuli on rhythmical masticatory movements in rabbits. *Archs oral Biol.* 16: 215-23

22 Luther, E.C., Arballo, J.C., Sala, N.L., and Cordero Funes, J.C. 1974. Suckling pressure in humans: relationship to oxytocin-reproducing reflex milk ejection. *J. appl. Physiol.* 36: 350-3

23 Maller, O., Kare, M.R., Welt, M., and Behrman, H. 1967. Movement of glucose and sodium chloride from the oropharyngeal cavity to the brain. *Nature* 213: 713-14

24 Marshall, J.F., Turner, B.H., and Teitelbaum, P. 1971. Sensory neglect produced by lateral hypothalamic damage. *Science* 174: 523-5

25 McGeer, P.L., and McGeer, E.G. 1973. Neurotransmitter synthetic enzymes. *Prog. Neurobiol.* 2: 71-117

26 McGinty, D., Epstein, A.N., and Teitelbaum, P. 1965. The contribution of oropharyngeal sensations to hypothalamic hyperphagia. *Animal Behav.* 13: 413-18

27 Meadows, J.C. 1973. Dysphagia in unilateral cerebral lesions. *J. Neurol. Neurosurg. Psychiat.* 36: 853-60

28 Menguy, R., Masters, Y.F., and Manzi, J. 1967. Characterization and partial purification of sialogastrone. *Surgery* 62: 891-8

29 Miles, T.S., and Dellow, P.G. 1971. The oral absorption of water. *Canad. J. Physiol. Pharmacol.* 49: 796-800

30 Mogenson, G.J., and Huang, Y.H. 1973. The neurobiology of motivated behavior. *Prog. Neurobiol.* 1: 53-83

31 Myers, R.D., and Martin, G.E. 1973. 6-OHDA lesions of the hypothalamus: interaction of aphagia, food palatability, set-point for weight regulation, and recovery of feeding. *Pharmacol. Biochem. Behav.* 1: 329-45

32 Nicolaïdis, S. 1968. Réponses des unités osmosensibles hypothalamiques aux stimulations salines et aqueuses de la langue. *C.R. Acad. Sci. (Paris).* Série D. 267: 2352-5

33 – 1969. Early systemic responses to orogastric stimulation in the regulation of food and water balance: functional and electrophysiological data. *Ann. N.Y. Acad. Sci.* 157: 1176-203

34 Phillips, A.G., and Fibiger, H.C. 1973. Substantia nigra: self-stimulation and post stimulation feeding. *Physiol. Psychol.* 1: 233-6

35 Routtenberg, A. 1972. Intracranial chemical injection and behaviour: a critical review. *Behav. Biol.* 7: 601-41

36 Rozkowska, E., and Fonberg, E. 1972. Impairment of salivary reflexes after lateral hypothalamic lesions in dogs. *Acta Neurobiol. Exp.* 32: 711–20

37 − 1973. Salivary reactions after ventromedial hypothalamic lesions in dogs. *Acta Neurobiol. Exp.* 33: 553–62

38 Russek, M. 1971. Hepatic receptors and the neurophysiological mechanisms controlling feeding behavior. *Neurosci. Res.* 4: 213–82

39 Rybakowa, M., Jakob-Dolezal, K., Knychalska-Karwan, Z., and Miezynski, M. 1973. The condition of the oral cavity in children with hypothalamo-hypophyseal insufficiency. *Czas. Stomat.* 26: 45–53

40 Samoilov, M.O. 1972. Efferent links of somatosensory regions of the neocortex with the hypothalamus in the cat. *Doklady Biol. Sci.* 204: 378–80

41 Scharer, P. 1971. Experimental bruxism in rabbits. *Helv. odont. Acta* 15: 54–7

42 Shapiro, M.M. 1960. Respondent salivary conditioning during operant lever pressing in dogs. *Science* 132: 619–20

43 Smith, D.A. 1972. Increased peri-oral responsiveness: a possible explanation for the switching of behavior observed during lateral hypothalamic stimulation. *Physiol. Behav.* 8: 617–21

44 Smith, G.P., Gibbs, J., and Young, R.C. 1974. Cholecystokinin and intestinal satiety in the rat. *Fed. Proc.* 33: 1146–9

45 Smith, M., and Duffy, M. 1957. Some physiological factors that regulate eating. *J. comp. Physiol. Psychol.* 50: 601–8

46 Sumi, T. 1972. Role of the pontine reticular formation in the neural organization of deglutition. *Jap. J. Physiol.* 22: 295–314

47 Thexton, A.J. 1973. Oral reflexes elicited by mechanical stimulation of palatal mucosa in the cat. *Archs oral Biol.* 18: 971–80

48 Voloschin, L.M., and Trammezani, J.H. 1973. The neural input of the milk ejection reflex in the hypothalamus. *Endocrinol.* 92: 973–83

49 Weiner, W.J., and Klawans, H.L. 1973. Lingual-facial-buccal movements in the elderly. I. Pathology and treatment. *J. Am. Geriat Soc.* 21: 314–17

50 Wenner, W.H., Douthitt, T.C., Burke, M.E., and Keenan, P.A. 1970. Observations on the regular recurrence of groups of spontaneous rhythmic oral activity in infants. In J.F. Bosma (ed.) *Second Symposium on Oral Sensation and Perception.* Springfield, Ill.: C.C. Thomas

51 Wolff, P.H. 1973. Natural history of sucking patterns in infant goats: a comparative study. *J. comp. Physiol. Psychol.* 84: 252–7

52 Wotman, S., Baer, L., Mandel, I.D., and Laragh, J.H. 1973. Salivary electrolytes, renin and aldosterone during sodium loading and depletion. *J. appl. Physiol.* 35: 322–4

53 Wyrwicka, W., and Chase, M.H. 1970. Projections from the buccal cavity to brain stem sites involved in feeding behavior. *Exp. Neurol.* 27: 512–19

54 Yaksh, T.L., and Myers, R.D. 1972. Neurohumoral substances released from hypothalamus of the monkey during hunger and satiety. *Am. J. Physiol.* 222: 503–15

55 Young, P.T. 1940. Reversal of food preference of the white rat through controlled pre-feeding. *J. gen. Psychol.* 22: 33–6

DISCUSSION

LUND   If the amount of brain development is so tied up with the mouth, one could argue that brain development would then depend very much upon the diet, and that animals which have to do a lot of work to get their food, e.g. carnivores would have more highly developed brains than animals which did not have to work so hard. I can immediately think of an exception, and that is the whale.

DELLOW   Yes, there is a most fascinating story about whales and dolphins as you probably know. There is no doubt that whales have the easiest time of all eating, particularly the filter feeders. The work of Lilly with respect to the dolphin is remarkable. The dolphin can reproduce human speech, and this phenomenon is probably related to brain size (e.g. J.C. Lilly, *Perspect. Biol. Med.* 6 [1963] : 246–55). Incidentally, the dolphin does not have much trouble eating.

THOMAS   You are aware, no doubt, of the work with split brains in which it has been shown that consciousness is related to the speech centres in the brain (e.g. J.C. Eccles, *Naturwissenschaften* 60 [1973]: 167-76). I wonder if you would be prepared to comment on that?

DELLOW   You are probably referring to the work on sidedness and speech. I believe that it has been shown that the left hemisphere is bigger in the newborn or during intrauterine life, the left side being the speech control side even in left-handed people (S.F. Witelson and W. Pallie, *Brain* 96 [1973]: 641–46). It has been suggested that the speech 'happening' or speech possibilities are inborn rather than just learned. Of course, there has to be a cortical development for the learning. Even if speech is controlled largely from the left hemisphere, the commissural input from the right hemisphere is obviously involved.

LUND   I think that the idea that one speech side is involved in consciousness arises from the fact that in the split-brain subject it is very difficult for one side of the brain to communicate with the other, so that although both sides of the brain are conscious, one side can only communicate with the other by means of gestures, etc.

DELLOW   Yes, there is quite an interesting dichotomy of function between
the two sides (R.W. Sperry, in F.O. Schmitt and F.G. Warden (eds.), *The
Neurosciences* [Massachusetts: M.I.T. Press, 1974]).

KAWAMURA   Dr Thomas, you have previously suggested that decerebrate
animals can chew. However, is there any coordinated function between tongue and mandible during chewing in those animals? I assume there is not; so
the higher brain centres would seem to be very important for this coordination.

THOMAS   We have not observed tongue movements during masticatory movements.

LUND   In our experiments involving stimulation of the descending motor
pathways (the corticobular tracts, and the brain stem after decerebration) we
cut the trigeminal nerves and we could see rhythmical activity in the facial
and in the tongue muscles (J.P. Lund, PHD thesis, Univ. Western Ontario
[1971]). If the hypoglossal nerve is cut, rhythmical movements of the facial
muscles occur without movements of the mandible or tongue. It would seem
that the basic coordination of these different muscle groups is achieved within
the brain stem.

MATTHEWS   Dr Thomas, how long have you kept decerebrate rats alive? Do
they make any attempt to eat, or search for and consume food on their own,
or do you have to maintain them by active feeding?

THOMAS   We have worked only on acute decerebrate animals, but Woods has
kept them alive for about 30 days (R. Woods, *J. Neurophysiol.* 27 [1964] :
635-44). In these animals there is no motivation to eat.

MATTHEWS   They chew food, but it has to be placed in the mouth first?

THOMAS   Yes. There is a similar effect with regard to coitus.

MATTHEWS   How did you actually stimulate chewing?

THOMAS   We stimulated the oral cavity and also depressed the mandible.

KAWAMURA   From the point of view of afferent input, we know that there
are few muscle spindles in the jaw-opening muscles. Probably the periodontal
receptors serve as a source of exteroceptive information, not proprioceptive,
so that when the periodontal receptors are stimulated jaw opening is induced.
This is an avoidance reflex. I am trying to emphasize the apparent function of
the Golgi tendon organ, and perhaps we can talk about this later in the symposium. To get back to coordination, we cannot speak while we chew, and we
cannot chew while we speak. So we must have a very finely coordinated
switch mechanism at work here.

DELLOW   Your findings (e.g. Y. Kawamura and A. Kamada, *J. dent. Res.* 46
[1967] : 452) interested me because the mandibular movements did switch
from vocalization to chewing.

KAWAMURA With regard to feeding behaviour, chewing movements may be induced when the feeding centre in the lateral hypothalamus is excited. What is the relationship between the cortical jaw motor areas and the feeding centre with regard to chewing?

DELLOW There are anatomical relationships. However, one of the mechanisms coming to light in the biochemical study of nervous tissue is that long dopaminergic pathways that go *through* the hypothalamus (as opposed to starting and stopping there) may be implicated. I think the hypothalamus has to be involved because one can take samples out of the hypothalamus of a hungry monkey and inject them into another monkey, causing it to eat (Yaksh and Myers, 1972). The question is, are the substances produced coming from a source here, or do they come from the pathways *en passant*. As you know, there is a 'nightmare' of structures in this area. Certainly stimulation of catecholaminergic pathways, or an imbalance between cholinergic and dopaminergic systems can cause chewing-like movements too. One of these pathways goes straight through the hypothalamus (U. Ungerstedt, *Neurosci. Res.* 5 [1973] 73-96), and is represented in Figure 3.

SESSLE Dr Lund, what is the rate of the rhythmic mouth opening movements that you see?

LUND The rate varies from 1/sec to about 5/sec, depending on stimulation rate.

SESSLE So you are getting facilitation.

THOMAS In our studies the cyclic movements are from 3 to 5 cycles/sec.

DELLOW We have been delivering a biochemical stimulus to the striatum, and when combined with jaw opening, the two together cause a rhythmical movement of about 3-4 cycles/sec.

ROYDHOUSE There are some other interesting observations that have been made about rhythms. For example, people who are unable to speak because of brain injuries are quite capable of singing, the rhythm apparently being able to evoke words.

DELLOW Yes. There is also a lot of work being done on accent rhythms in language at present. These demonstrate differences in the emphasis on syllables (R. Netsell, in F. Minifie, T. Nixon, and F. Williams (eds.), *Normal Aspects of Speech, Hearing and Language* [New Jersey: Prentice-Hall, 1973]). In Japanese I believe the accent is on every syllable, whereas in English it is on every few syllables; that is why our verse is so pleasant to listen to.

ROYDHOUSE Taking this a bit further, it has been suggested that there are in-built patterns of grammatical construction which are common to the human race and expressed by people independent of their upbringing (N. Chomsky, *Studies on Semantics in Generative Grammar* [The Hague: Mouton, 1972]). When you learn a language you do not necessarily learn the logic of it.

I have observed that the only pain which will stop people from talking is trigeminal neuralgia: patients are unable to speak during an attack, and one has the impression that they are also unable to think.

DELLOW Yes. However, a lot of patients will vocalize at the beginning of an attack.

SESSLE Dr Dellow, you mentioned also the topic of suckling. Do you think there is any ontogenetic or phylogenetic evidence for mastication being just a follow-on of suckling? For example, in the human, suckling appears first and it involves tongue and coordinated jaw movements. After a time, when the dentition appears, breast feeding gradually decreases and mastication begins. Thus there is already a basis for coordinated tongue and jaw movements.

DELLOW That would be my interpretation exactly. I also suspect that the intrinsic rhythms are there for speech as well.

SESSLE It seems that the same muscles are involved in lapping, sucking, and mastication, and that the coordinating mechanisms could essentially be a natural progression from one to the rest. Of course, a change in sensory feedback probably occurs with mastication, e.g. from the teeth.

DELLOW As the baby is learning to masticate he is also learning to speak. There is much interest shown these days in 'baby babbling,' and the feeling is that rather than being just 'gobbledegook,' it could be quite important (N.S. Rees, *Brit. J. Dis. Comm.* 7 [1972]: 17-23).

LUND Although there may be some common mechanisms involved in suckling and mastication, there are some differences. For example, in suckling there is very active opening of the jaws, with the development of reduced pressure in the mouth, whereas mastication is mainly an activity of the jaw-closing muscles.

SESSLE But activity in the jaw-closing muscles is also a very important part of suckling (e.g. J.F. Bosma, *Oral Sensation and Perception* [Springfield, Ill.: Thomas, 1967]). The reason why I brought the subject up is because it may be involved, for example, in tongue-thrust swallowing; the tongue may not lose its ability to come forward, as in suckling. This may have some clinical significance.

DELLOW A goat's tail will wag, and kittens will paw at the same rate as the animal sucks (H.F.R. Prechtl, *Experentia* 8 [1952]: 220-1; Wolff, 1973). One cannot help but think that perhaps the spinal cord pattern generator is linked to work as well.

THOMAS Yes, the administration of dopamine and clonidine has been shown to produce walking movements in mesencephalic cats (H. Forssberg and S. Grillner, *Brain Res.* 50 [1973]: 184-6).

Interactions of alimentary and upper respiratory tract reflexes

A.T. STOREY

The two reflexes under scrutiny at this conference are both alimentary reflexes. Most of the action in both mastication and swallowing takes place in the mouth, the biological objective of this action being mechanical degradation of the food ingested and its conveyance to the stomach. The mouth also plays a transient role in respiratory functions. Mouth breathing occurs on the occasion of vigorous exercise, with nasal or nasopharyngeal obstruction, in speech and singing, and in snoring. Swallowing activity also engages the pharynx – a region which serves an obligatory respiratory and alimentary role. It is in the pharynx that the two tracts cross (see Fig. 1). Above the pharynx the airway is dorsal to the alimentary tract – below the pharynx the airway is ventral. This crossing has greatly complicated the organization of upper alimentary and airway reflexes as will be obvious a little later in this presentation. How much simpler if the upper respiratory and alimentary tracts had retained a constant relationship throughout the head and neck. How did this crossing evolve? The ventral position of the airway was laid down when the tetrapods (which include modern amphibians, reptiles, birds, and mammals) evolved a ventral airway and lungs while the ancestors of living fishes evolved a dorsal lung position. Opting for the early teleost orientation would have obviated a pharyngeal crossing on the acquisition of a nasal airway to subserve olfaction. The other alternative would have been a nose under the chin!

An important feature of the respiratory pharynx is the anatomical structure which forms its ventral wall. We all realize it is the base of the tongue. Remember then that the tongue, while manipulating the bolus in mastication, is also serving as the anterior wall of a functioning pharyngeal airway. During swallowing the tongue briefly relinquishes this respiratory role to propel the bolus, piston-like, into a pharynx which also momentarily relinquishes its respiratory function.

Let us now turn our attention to the reflexes of the upper airway and alimentary tract. Let us look at some examples of airway reflexes. I have

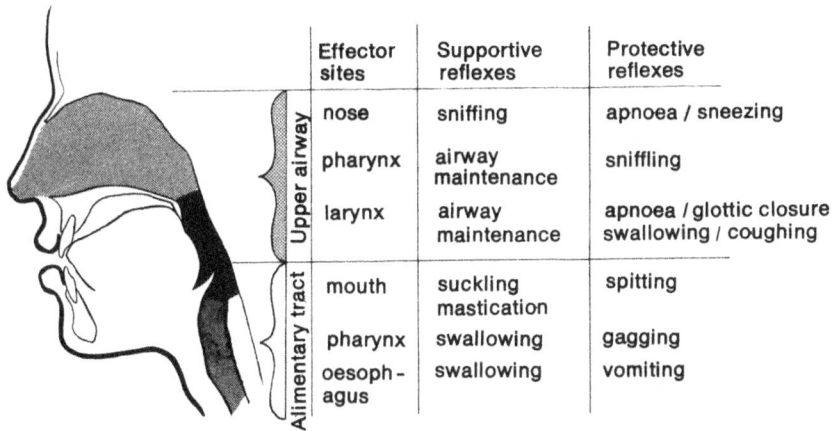

	Effector sites	Supportive reflexes	Protective reflexes
Upper airway	nose	sniffing	apnoea / sneezing
	pharynx	airway maintenance	sniffling
	larynx	airway maintenance	apnoea / glottic closure swallowing / coughing
Alimentary tract	mouth	suckling mastication	spitting
	pharynx	swallowing	gagging
	oesoph-agus	swallowing	vomiting

FIGURE 1 Effector sites giving rise to supportive and protective reflexes of the upper airway and alimentary tract. The upper airway is indicated in the figure to the left with light stipple, the alimentary tract with no stipple. Note that in the pharynx the two tracts cross (heavy stipple).

grouped both respiratory and alimentary reflexes into supportive and protective reflexes. Supportive reflexes are concerned with obtaining air and food; protective reflexes with preventing entry into, or expelling harmful materials from, the airway or alimentary tract. Some of these reflexes are listed in Figure 1. Supportive reflexes of the upper airway include sniffing and airway maintenance. Sniffing in macrosmatic animals aids in the finding of food; reflexes maintaining the airway regulate the size of both the pharyngeal and laryngeal airways. The size of the pharyngeal airway is regulated by reflexes regulating tongue and mandibular position and to some degree head posture. Protective reflexes of the upper airway are numerous. Nasal irritants produce apnoea to prevent further inhalation, or sneezing to eliminate the offending substance. Sniffling (aspiration reflex) moves nasopharyngeal irritants into the pharynx for swallowing. Apnoea and glottic closure protect the larynx from invasion. Swallowing removes small quantities of liquid material from the laryngeal isthmus, and coughing larger quantities of liquids or particulate matter.

Supportive reflexes of the upper alimentary tract include suckling, mastication, and swallowing: protective reflexes that come to mind are spitting, gagging, and vomiting. Note that each effector site possesses both supportive and protective reflexes. As a general rule there is a hierarchical structure to these reflexes, with protective reflexes taking precedence over supportive reflexes and airway reflexes superseding alimentary tract reflexes. This illustrates the complexity of reflex organization alluded to earlier. I do not know whether a protective reflex in one effector site can displace a protective reflex in the other: stimuli eliciting protective reflexes in both tracts at the same time must be exceedingly rare. All protective reflexes supersede airway supportive reflexes - for example, swallowing inhibits respiration. Airway supportive reflexes override alimentary supportive reflexes - for example, airway maintenance overrides suckling, mastication, and swallowing.

Note that I have categorized swallowing as both an airway protective reflex and an alimentary supportive reflex. The idea that swallowing is an airway protective reflex may be new to some. Kahn (1903) first hinted at this possibility and I advanced the hypothesis after I found that laryngeal stimulation by water was a most effective means of initiating swallowing in the decerebrate animal (Storey, 1968a). It had been known for many years that electrical stimulation of the superior laryngeal nerve (SLN) was more effective in eliciting swallowing than stimulation of the glossopharyngeal nerve (GPN) or the trigeminal nerve. All three nerves innervate areas that can give rise to swallowing. The preferential effect of SLN stimulation could be due to excitation of fewer inhibitory fibres or a larger population of excitatory fibres. The former possibility seems more likely since Sinclair (1975), working in my laboratory, has found that the GPN fibres (1-6 μ in diameter) most likely to initiate swallowing, on the basis of single unit responses to the adequate stimulus, are as abundant in the GPN as in the SLN. This predominance of the SLN in swallowing is also true for humans. Neurological studies by Fay (1927), Ballantine et al. (1954), Uihlein, Love, and Corbin (1955), and Chawla and Falconer (1967) on patients suffering from glossopharyngeal neuralgia in whom GPNs were transected bilaterally showed that swallowing was not impaired by these transections.

The concept that swallowing is primarily initiated from the pharynx is invalid. The larynx (including the epiglottis) is the major site of initiation of swallowing. What function does the laryngeal swallow serve? I think it serves to guard the larynx from invasion by saliva and liquid bolus residues. It probably removes airway secretions which dribble down from above or are wafted up from the trachea by the action of the ciliated epithelium.

So far I have catalogued a number of respiratory and alimentary reflexes occupying the regions participating in mastication and swallowing in order to demonstrate that each region is capable of giving rise to a number of reflexes which are ordered in hierarchical fashion. Some of these reflexes such as mastication, swallowing, coughing, or gagging are complex enough when viewed in isolation, but when their interactions are considered the control system looks formidable. Obviously there is another order of integration that deter-

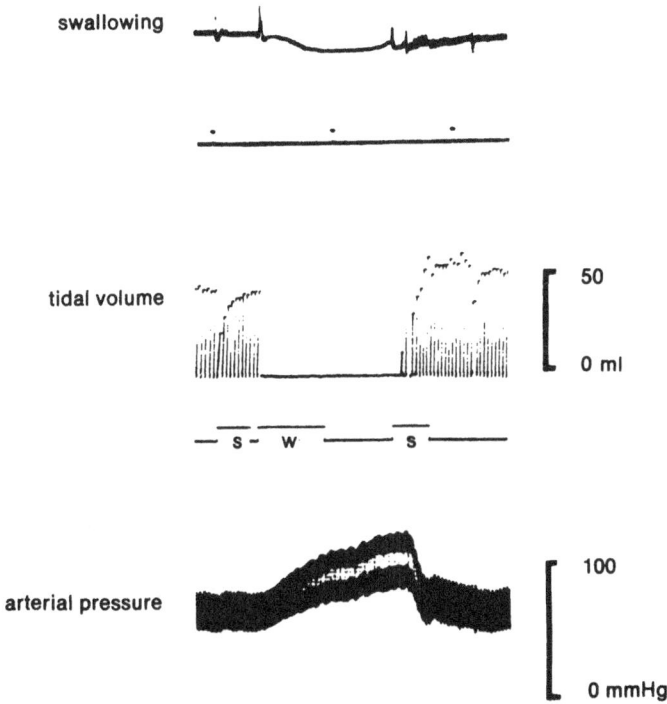

FIGURE 2 Alimentary, respiratory and cardiovascular responses in a lamb six hours old to water stimulation of the larynx. The three data traces from top to bottom depict swallows (large upgoing spikes), tidal volume in inspiration, and femoral arterial pressure. The time markers on the second channel are one minute apart and the upward displacements of the base line in channel four indicate saline(s) or water (w) flowing through the larynx from the trachea into the mouth. In the lamb water stimulation of the larynx produces apnoea as long as the water remains in the larynx; in older lambs water stimulation results in variable reductions in tidal volume.

mines which reflexes will occupy the stage at a particular moment in time. Some reflexes can perform together, for example mastication and airway maintenance; others such as swallowing and airway maintenance are incompatible.

What determines whether an intrusion into the larynx is going to result in apnoea, glottic closure, swallowing, or coughing? In the normal adult animal any detectable stimulus will produce apnoea of variable duration. The apnoeic reflex is much more powerful at certain stages of development. In a young lamb of susceptible breed, water stimulation of the larynx produces apnoea (Fig. 2) as long as the water stimulus remains (Storey and Johnson, 1975). The animal will die if the water stimulus is not removed. On the other hand, an older lamb may be made only partially apnoeic by the identical stimulus. Water is an effective stimulus to swallowing in the older lamb. Does the swallowing remove the water from the larynx and thereby remove the deadly effect of the water? Or is the lamb maturing and thereby becoming less vulnerable to the water stimulation. I interject this feature of the apnoeic response to demonstrate that many of these reflexes change with maturation. Suckling is an example of a supportive reflex which also attenuates with maturation. Any detectable stimulus in the larynx will produce apnoea of variable duration. A small quantity of water will result in apnoea and swallowing. A weak mechanical stimulus will result in apnoea and glottic closure while a stronger mechanical stimulus will result in coughing. By what mechanism is the appropriate reflex elicited? Sometimes the effective stimuli for two reflexes occur at the same time: when they are incompatible as swallowing and coughing, how is the inappropriate reflex inhibited?

Some insight can be gained by looking at the discharge of a superficial laryngeal receptor to the stimuli which produce the above responses. The temporal relationship of action potentials recorded from a single tactile unit located in the mucosa overlying the thyroarytenoid muscle of a cat (Storey, 1968b) is illustrated in Figure 3B, C, and D. A weak mechanical stimulus produces the discharge B in one such unit, while a strong mechanical stimulus produces the discharge C, and water the discharge D. These discharges are reproduced with the response produced by the same stimulus in the innervated larynx indicated to the right of the arrows. A monotonic pulse train of 30 impulses/sec – the optimal frequency for eliciting swallowing by electrical stimulation of the SLN – is provided for comparison. The high-frequency discharge would appear to give rise to coughing but the lower frequency discharges may give rise to either glottic closure or swallowing. Frequency of discharge alone cannot account for the appropriate response. Although water excites only superficial receptors, mechanical stimulation excites deeper receptors (or higher threshold superficial receptors).

Since slightly higher voltages are required to elicit coughing rather than swallowing on SLN stimulation (Storey, 1968c) and local anaesthetic abolishes coughing before swallowing (Sinclair, unpublished observations), fibres smaller than those eliciting swallowing are excited in coughing. Our hypothesis is that low-frequency activity limited to superficial receptors initiates swallowing (hatched squares in the upper right portion of Fig. 4). Movement of the stimulus makes it more effective – perhaps sequential activation of superficial receptors is an important factor (lower right portion of Fig. 4). We speculate that for glottic closure and coughing another population of receptors is added (the solid squares in the left half of Fig. 4). Perhaps low-frequency discharges in one or both populations determines glottic closure whereas higher frequencies

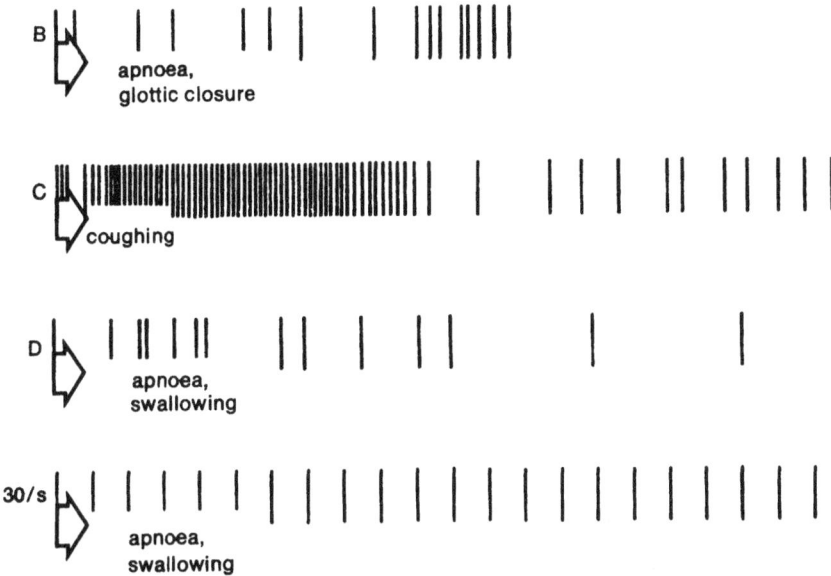

FIGURE 3   The temporal relationship of discharges in a single sensory fibre of the superior laryngeal nerve of the cat to B (light contact), C (pressure) and D (water) applied to the fibre's sensory field on the laryngeal mucosa overlying the ipsilateral thyroarytenoid muscle. In B the discharge continued as long as contact was maintained; in C the discharge continued after stimulation had ceased. In D the duration of the stimulus is difficult to specify since one or two drops of water were dribbled over the receptive field. A monotonic signal of 30 impulses/sec, which is the optimal frequency for eliciting swallowing by electrical stimulation, is provided for comparison. In innervated larynges the stimulus giving rise to impulse trains similar to B initiate apnoea and glottic closure, the stimulus for C coughing, and the stimulus for D apnoea and swallowing.

trigger coughing. Both the spectrum of receptor types excited as well as the frequency of discharge of those receptors could account for the appropriate protective reflex.

Such a model says nothing about how these inputs interact centrally to initiate the appropriate response – or to inhibit inappropriate responses. The two receptor populations proposed could exert facilitatory or inhibitory effects either postsynaptically or presynaptically. Sessle (1973a) has shown that SLN primary afferents can exert both facilitatory and inhibitory effects on second-order neurones. These afferents can depolarize other SLN primary afferents which may be an indication of presynaptic inhibition. Sessle (1973b) has shown similar effects produced by trigeminal and glossopharyngeal afferents suggesting that the appropriate elicitation of a response may not be determined exclusively in the region which gives rise to the reflex.

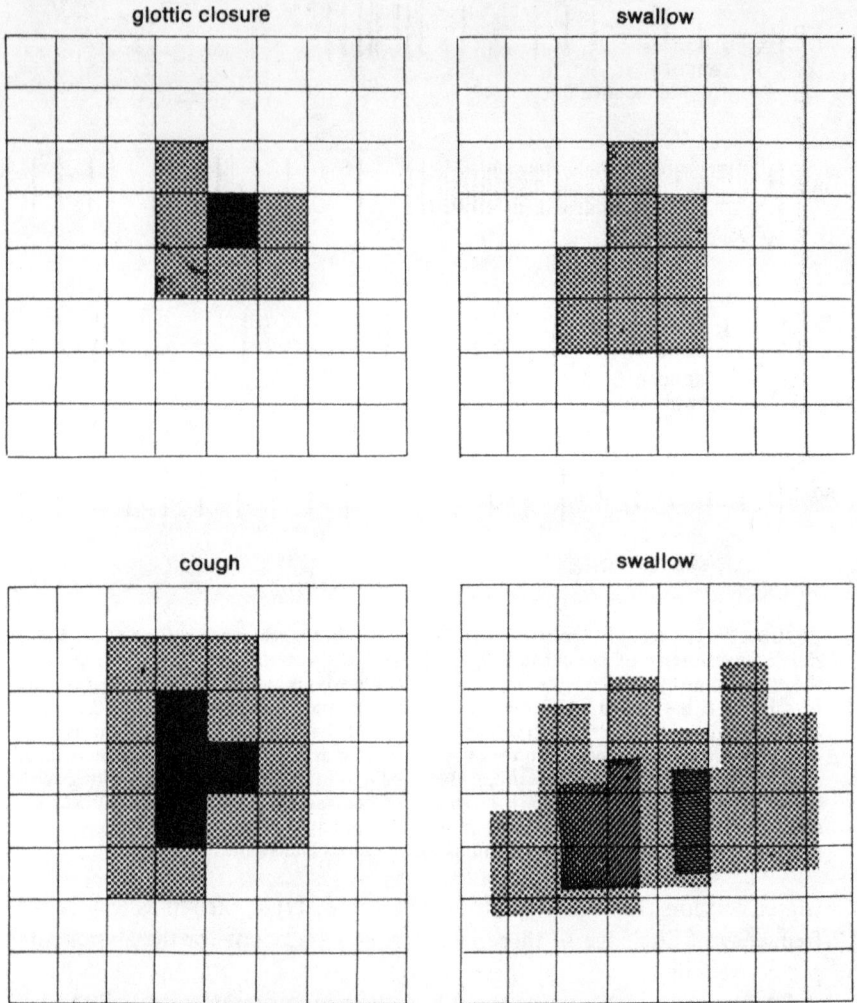

FIGURE 4 Hypothetical excitation patterns of laryngeal receptors giving rise to laryngeal reflexes. Each square depicts the receptive field of one sensory unit. Solid squares represent fields innervated by fibres smaller than those innervating fields represented by the stippled squares (solid squares may also indicate receptors firing at a higher frequency than surrounding receptors). According to this scheme, swallowing is elicited by one population of receptors firing at low frequencies (upper right). Movement of the stimulus enhances swallow elicitation (lower right). Glottic closure and swallowing may result from stimulation of two populations of receptors of high (solid) and low (stippled) threshold supplied by very small and small-sized fibres respectively. Alternatively these reflexes may arise from stimulation of similar receptors at high (solid square) and low (stippled square) frequencies.

These inputs also appear to set the stage for swallowing in appropriate motoneurones. Sumi (1969) has shown that repetitive SLN stimulation partially depolarizes hypoglossal neurones before they fire as part of the swallowing synergy. Although these peripheral inputs have been considered in relationship to the initiation of reflexes they probably play a role in modulating ongoing reflex activity. This aspect of mastication and swallowing will be examined closely during this conference. However, any feedback on mastication and swallowing must in part be directed at reflexes maintaining and protecting the airway.

This leads me to interactions between specific alimentary and respiratory tract reflexes: between mastication and airway maintenance, swallowing and protection of the airway, and mastication and swallowing. I have already indicated that the anterior wall of the pharyngeal airway is created by the base of the tongue. During mastication and prior to swallowing, the mouth is sealed off from the pharynx by a barrier formed by tongue contact with the soft palate and the faucial pillars (Bosma, 1957). During mastication the tongue must serve two masters – while the anterior two-thirds of the tongue is concerned with bolus manipulation and tasting, the posterior third is concerned with airway maintenance. Perhaps this duality of roles should not be a surprise considering the common embryological origins of the base of the tongue and the pharynx.

Whereas mastication interacts with supportive reflexes of the airway, swallowing interacts with protective reflexes of the airway. Apnoea and glottic closure persist for the duration of the swallowing. Elevation of the larynx appears to occur only as a part of the swallowing reflex. Apnoea and glottic closure appear to be under the direct control of the swallowing centre. Apnoea and glottic closure can, of course, occur independently of swallowing. Although feedback does not appear to play a role in swallowing in the adult animal, Sumi (1975) has suggested recently that it may be significant in the young animal.

The infantile swallow is characterized by tongue thrusting. Is the tongue thrusting the result of inadequate feedback in an immature regulatory mechanism? Or is it a mechanism to maintain the airway where the tongue is too large for the jaws? This seems unlikely, since the pharynx relinquishes its airway function during swallowing. Perhaps it is the maintenance of an adequate passage for transmission of the bolus. Why then the need for protrusion of the tongue with a liquid bolus where the minimal luminal requirements are only 3-4 mm (Bosma, 1957)? Is it a retention of the infantile mechanism for effecting an anterior mouth seal before the teeth erupt – or is it a vestige of infantile suckling? Does tongue thrusting cause anterior open bite or is it the result of anterior posturing of the tongue to maintain an adequate pharyngeal airway? Perhaps the protracted tongue in postural position does the damage and the tongue thrust is an adaptation to the open bite. Answers to the questions posed above are needed to establish a more rational treatment of tongue thrusting.

Finally, I would like to make a few observations on the interaction between mastication and swallowing. After a certain number of masticatory cycles or chews on a degradable bolus, swallowing ensues. What determines the number of chews, i.e. the swallowing threshold? Dahlberg (1946) and Yurkstas (1951) have demonstrated that it is not particle size since no compensation is made for an inadequate dentition – the subject swallows larger particles. The initial expectation would be that swallowing occurs when the bolus particles are degraded to a certain size. This expectation produces a number of paradoxes. First, the regions of the mouth best equipped to monitor particle size, e.g. the teeth, tongue, and palate, do not give rise to swallowing. Secondly, as the particles are degraded they would be less likely to excite these receptors. Thirdly, the oropharyngeal sites which do give rise to swallowing are covered by the tongue during mastication. As Pommerenke (1928) has shown, these most reflexogenic sites are the faucial pillars and the posterior pharyngeal wall. How then is swallowing initiated during mastication?

Mention was made earlier that the epiglottis and larynx are the most reflexogenic sites for swallowing. I speculate that it is the aqueous vehicle of the bolus and/or saliva dribbling down over the back of the tongue onto the epiglottis that triggers off the swallow. Since the epiglottis has a common embryological origin with the pharynx, it is possible to think of the laryngeal swallow serving both an alimentary and a respiratory function. If this is the mechanism for determining swallowing threshold, one would expect the rapidity of swallowing to be proportional to the fluidity of the bolus. This fits the facts. We swallow liquids at once and succulent foods very quickly. The swallowing threshold for other foods might be a function of how rapidly they stimulated salivary flow as a result of gustatory or mechanical stimulation.

In summary, I would like to emphasize that mastication and swallowing utilize anatomical components of the airway, namely, base of tongue and pharynx and therefore these two reflexes must be integrated with respiratory reflexes. Respiratory reflexes and protective reflexes will pre-empt these two alimentary reflexes when the occasion arises. I think it important to remember as well that the primary region for elicitation of swallowing is the epiglottis and rostral larynx and not the pharynx. Swallowing elicited here serves both alimentary and respiratory functions.

REFERENCES

Ballantine, H.T., Talbert, R., Currens, J.H., and Cohen, M.E. 1954. Studies of sensation, circulation and respiration after bilateral glossopharyngeal rhizotomy. *Trans. Am. Neurol. Assoc.* 79: 69–72

Bosma, J.F. 1957. Deglutition: pharyngeal stage. *Physiol. Rev.* 37: 275–300

Chawla, J.C., and Falconer, M.A. 1967. Glossopharyngeal and vagal neuralgia. *Brit. Med. J.* 3: 529–31

Dahlberg, B. 1946. The masticatory habits. An analysis of the number of chews when consuming food. *J. dent. Res.* 25: 67–72

Fay, T. 1927. Observation and results from intracranial section of the glossopharyngeal and vagus nerves in man. *J. Neuropathol. exp. Neurol.* 8: 11–123

Kahn, R.H. 1903. Studien uber den Schluckreflex. *Arch. Physiol. Suppl.* 27: 386–426

Pommerenke, W.T. 1928. A study of the sensory areas eliciting the swallowing reflex. *Am. J. Physiol.* 84: 36–41

Sessle, B.J. 1973a. Excitatory and inhibitory inputs to single neurones in the solitary tract nucleus and adjacent reticular formation. *Brain Res.* 53: 319–31

– 1973b. Presynaptic excitability changes induced in single laryngeal primary afferent fibres. *Brain Res.* 53: 333–42

Sinclair, W.J. 1975. *The pharyngeal plexus: an anatomical, histological and single unit analysis in the cat.* PHD Thesis, Univ. of Toronto

Storey, A.T. 1968a. Laryngeal initiation of swallowing. *Exp. Neurol.* 20: 359–65

– 1968b. A functional analysis of sensory units innervating epiglottis and larynx. *Exp. Neurol.* 20: 366–83

– 1968c. Discharge parameters initiating swallowing and coughing. *Proc. 46th Gen. Session IADR*, p. 85, Abstract 190

Storey, A.T., and Johnson, P. 1975. Laryngeal water receptors initiating apnea in the lamb. *Exp. Neurol.* 47: 42–55

Sumi, T. 1969. Synaptic potentials of hypoglossal motoneurons and their relation to reflex deglutition. *Jap. J. Physiol.* 19: 68–79

– 1975. Coordination of neural organization of respiration and deglutition; its change with postnatal maturation. In J.F. Bosma and J. Showacre (eds.), *Development of Upper Respiratory Form and Function: Implications for Sudden and Unexpected Infant Death.* Bethesda: D.H.E.W. in press

Uihlein, A., Love, J.G., and Corbin, K.B. 1955. Intracranial section of the glossopharyngeal nerve. Sensory changes observed postoperatively. *Arch. Neurol. Psychiat.* 74: 320–4

Yurkstas, A. 1951. Compensation for inadequate mastication. *Brit. dent. J.* 91: 261–2

DISCUSSION

LUND   You mentioned differences between new-born and older lambs. Is this behaviour consistent?

STOREY   It depends upon the breed to some degree. Some animals are more susceptible than others. If you take the same breed, then the pattern is quite consistent.

LUND   Apart from explaining the phenomenon as a maturational effect, could it be that there are differences in the type of secretions present in the young and older animals?

STOREY   I am not quite sure what function these secretions of the larynx would have if they were not washed away. I think that they might have a protective function. However, when you flow the stimulus through you eventually wash away most of the secretions, and the response is still only momentary in the older animals. If you have a derangement in the area, the situation may be different. Lately, I have been looking at the possibility that inflammation and sensitization in the larynx may facilitate the apnoeic response in the older animal, and indeed this seems to be the case. We speculate that this is related to the release of histamine.

LUND   I agree that the different reflex responses you have described may be due to differences in the receptor types you are stimulating. Could they not also be related to the numbers of afferent units you stimulate?

STOREY   The problem is in differentiating between the very light tactile stimulus and the water stimulus. The water stimulus is likely to activate quite a few receptors, whereas the tactile would activate relatively few. The stimulus for coughing would activate a fair number. If you look at Sinclair's work using differential anaesthetization of the superior laryngeal nerve, as the anaesthetic starts to take effect, the cough disappears first, and leaves swallowing intact. The way it comes back is appropriately reversed as the anaesthetic wears off, which tends to argue that it is not just the number but rather a difference in the population of fibres excited in each case.

LUND   Perhaps one could approach the problem by cutting down the nerve and stimulating the various branches.

STOREY   Yes, I have done that (Storey, 1968c). I have fractionated the nerve, but you soon reach a point where further division becomes very difficult. Until that point you can elicit the three responses from the split nerves. These are rather crude experiments where I have just kept taking pieces off the nerve to see if I can sustain a reflex. You can do this until you get down to about 1/10th of the original nerve. There is an additional problem here in that one would conceivably be damaging more of one sort of fibre than another. |

DELLOW   Before birth I understand the lungs are full of amniotic fluid, and that the foetus can and does swallow a large amount of it. What is the change that occurs with sudden lung expansion?

STOREY   The foetus not only swallows, but also 'respires' or breathes amniotic fluid. This has been clearly shown for the human foetus as well (G. Dawes et al., *J. Physiol. (Lond.)* 220 [1972]: 119-43). How much of this occurs, one does not know. It is curious that, when it happens, it does so during REM sleep or the equivalent of it in the foetus.

DELLOW   What interests me is how the fluid all of a sudden causes a protective reflex to be evoked.

STOREY   The argument has been, until the demonstration that there are these movements within the foetus, that the amniotic fluid excites the laryngeal receptors and prevents the animal from respiring, and that when he is born, the stimulus is removed and he then starts respiring. This now does not seem to be the case. If we look at the electrolyte content of amniotic fluid it is isotonic, so therefore it may behave like saline and we would not expect it to have an effect. There are some who believe that the laryngeal protective reflex against water is just one of a larger area of protection against water. For example, in the young rabbit water stimulation in the nose has the same effect as water in the larynx of the young lamb. The kitten and the guinea pig on the other hand seem to be mixed, both nasal and laryngeal sites being capable of inhibiting respiration. There are some who believe that this may have some relationship to drowning in the adult: that death may result from reflex respiratory inhibition rather than from asphyxia caused by the inhalation of water.

DELLOW   At what phase of respiration does the apnoeic period begin? It seems rather important, because if fluid causes it, the next breath should not be inspiration.

SUMI   I would like to point out that if perfume is introduced into the nose of the experimental animal, respiration ceases in the inspiratory position. If you increase the amount of perfume, respiration ceases in the expiratory position.

STOREY   The stimulus becomes offensive then?

SUMI   Yes. In addition, the level of anaesthesia appears to be critical.

STOREY   I take your point. The animals I spoke about were anaesthetized with chloralose. I have not looked very closely at when arrest occurred, partly because we were interested in the sudden infant death syndrome (SIDS) and it did not seem to matter much where they stopped breathing. More important was the fact that they stopped.

MATTHEWS   When you were recording afferent activity, were all the fibres which responded to water also responsive to mechanical stimulation?

STOREY   We did not examine it carefully in the lambs because we did not expose the larynx. In the cat there were a large number which responded to both (Storey, 1968b). The whole water receptor story is getting a lot of attention at present. The gustatory physiologists are looking at it closely, and they are inclined to think that the taste buds are probably the source of lingual water responses. Recently, Harding and Leek (*J. Physiol. (Lond.)* 222 [1972]: 139-40P) have shown that scraping the superficial mucosa of the gut wall eliminates the chemo response but not the mechano response of duodenal water receptors. It looks as if the units are branched. At least the gustatory physiologist will now acknowledge that some of the chemoreceptors are mechanosensitive. In addition they also recognize that water is not a neutral stimulus (L.M. Bartoshuk et al., *Science* 171 [1971]: 699-701). This has often been assumed in the past where water has commonly been used as the rinse in gustatory experiments. Moreover, those working on water receptors in the tongue also accept that water is not the only non-mechanical stimulus which will excite these receptors. For example, ammonium chloride is an active stimulant.

MATTHEWS   Have you had an opportunity to look at any of these other stimuli with regard to the apnoeic response?

STOREY   Yes. We know that acid will evoke it very powerfully, which raises the possibility that maybe this affords protection against the regurgitation of stomach contents. We have also looked at the effect of milk as well. It was suggested a long time ago that sudden infant death is due to sensitization to milk. Milk, in the unsensitized animal, will give a response halfway between water and isotonic saline. This fits in with its tonicity. In the guinea pig, sensitized to milk, there is a very powerful laryngeal response, more powerful than that to water. I do not think the effect is at the neural membrane. I think that probably what is happening is that the antigen-antibody reaction is releasing histamine (or other mediators) and the histamine is acting as the stimulus. We know that histamine is a very powerful stimulus to free nerve endings.

GREENWOOD   If you increase the tactile stimulus intensity you obtain a coughing response. Did you try increasing the area over which you applied the tactile stimulus?

STOREY   The area is an important factor. If you deliver a very large water stimulus in the experimental animal he does not swallow, he coughs. In this sense, the number of receptors excited is significant.

KAWAMURA   It seems that we are able to produce different reflex responses from stimulation of the same areas of the larynx. This poses the real physiological problem of how the central connections sort out the signals and produce the different response patterns.

STOREY   Quite so. What bothers me for example is why we do not gag with tongue contact in those sensitive areas initiating the reflex. It does not take much mechanical stimulation to produce a gag reflex.

SESSLE Obviously presynaptic inhibition is the answer! (Laughter).

DUBNER I would like to pursue this problem of different receptors initiating the various reflexes as opposed to the idea that it may be purely a summation effect. Do you know of any evidence that these reflexes could be initiated through a summation effect? Filling the larynx with a lot of water instead of a small amount could still excite a different receptor population.

STOREY No I do not. The difficulty, of course, is determining the number of fields being excited, particularly with water stimulation. These fields tend to be small.

KUBOTA To approach the question in another way, is there any evidence for different groups of discharge patterns in the afferents from the larynx when you use mechanical stimulation?

STOREY Occasionally in a small strand several units can be differentiated from each other. In the cat, mechanical stimulation of the laryngeal mucosa will activate superficial tactile-water units (low-threshold) or deeper pressure units (higher threshold). The adequate stimuli for apnoea, glottic closure, and swallowing excite only the superficial units. The adequate stimulus for coughing may involve the deeper units as well; it certainly elicits higher frequency activity in some of the tactile units.

HANNAM Where do we stand then at present with regard to the aetiology of SIDS?

STOREY There are a number of hypotheses. Maybe the answer to the question is that there is not one cause, but many. There are some who believe that the basic cause is an obstruction. This might take many forms, e.g. nasal obstruction in obligate nose breathers, the tongue falling back into the pharynx when reflexes which protect the airway for some reason give up. There are others who suggest that the chemoreceptors which are responsible for respiratory drive and regulation become turned off for some reason, and that the sleep state has something to do with it. People are looking at infants who have apnoeic episodes who are considered to be a high risk for SIDS. I think the encouraging thing is that hypotheses are being eliminated very rapidly. The emphasis now is on half a dozen. We just happen to be keen on the laryngeal one at the present (B.J. Sessle et al., *Canad. J. Physiol. Pharmacol.* 52 [1974]: 895-8; A.T. Storey and P. Johnson, 1975).

GOLDBERG As you mentioned, there is considerable interest at the moment in the various sleep stages and their relationship to SIDS. Colleagues of mine at UCLA are presently recording unit activity from the larynx of 5-10 day-old kittens with the idea that laryngospasm, in association with sleep stages, is implicated in the condition. Some interesting things may come out of this with regard to presynaptic effects, feedback from the area, and the resulting patterns of muscle contraction.

ROYDHOUSE From your hierarchical organization of reflexes it is probable that tongue position is more important than jaw position.

STOREY You have to look at the tongue, mandible, and inframandibular region as a functional unit, especially with regard to the maintenance of the airway and posture. When we are talking about the rest position of the mandible we ought to be considering the tongue, and the rest of the system. They belong together because of the dictates of the airway.

ROYDHOUSE Yes, Fish (*Brit. dent. J.* 116 [1964] : 149-59) suggests that the rest position of the mandible depends on the tongue. Incidentally, more than half the patients I see with mandibular dysfunction have swollen submandibular glands. This could have some effect on mandibular posture.

Chairman's Summary

N.R. THOMAS

The oral cavity participates in a large number of physiological activities including prehension, gustation, salivation, digestion, mastication, lapping, suckling, stereognosis, vocalization, water balance (thirst), and reflection of the organism's emotional set. Dr Dellow has presented a convincing case in support of the theory that these activities originated with, and have evolved from, the food and water needs of the organism. He has further advocated the corollary of this: namely that food is the most important influence in determining the organization of the brain and the behaviour that the brain organization dictates. Homer W. Smith (1953) expressed this in a poignant and intuitive statement: 'Without the predatory powers of jaws and teeth and the possibility of swift and accurate pursuit of prey there would have been no evolution of the sense organs of smell, sight and hearing, of elaborate muscular coordination, of prevision of how to get from here to there and the possible consequences of the transit - in short, there would have been no centralization of the nervous system such as ultimately produced the brain, and the earth would never have known the phenomenon of consciousness at least of an order superior to that of the lobster, scorpion or butterfly.' Eccles (1973), drawing from the split brain studies of Sperry (1968), argued that consciousness, as the ultimate function of the brain, is associated with the dominant hemisphere only owing to the development within it of an oral communication or speech centre. Sperry's work clearly establishes that the minor hemisphere devoid of speech function is also deprived of conscious experience.

'The need for oxygen is even more urgent than that for food, so urgent in fact that the nervous organization allows no room for compromise. The action of the respiratory centres like the act of breathing itself is so automatic that it is a bore. We cannot choose whether or what or how to breathe. But with eating, how different it is!' (Young, 1968). Where there is no choice there can be no learning. This was inherent in Dr Lund's question. The capacity for choice on the part of the whale (cetacea) has permitted successful

radiation into a great variety of diversified sublines such as the giant whale-
bone food-strainers (which also develop teeth that fail to erupt), the big-
toothed whales specialized to feed on deep-sea cuttlefish, the carnivorous
killer whales attacking other marine animals, and the porpoises and dolphins
specialized for fish eating. The background for all learning systems is that the
organism has the capacity to take any one of two or more actions in response
to a given stimulus situation. If the organism does not have the ability to recognize, to remember, and to analyse, then its capacity for response to a
stimulus situation provided by the environment is limited. There appears to
be unanimous agreement that the 'choice' associated with food intake provided the stimulus for brain development.

The enormous list of activities performed by the oral cavity thus implies a
complex coordinating mechanism or brain. Accordingly the main nerve supplying the oral cavity (the trigeminal) is unique both for its tremendous size
and for the number and complexity of its interconnections with other cranial
nuclei including the nerve most closely associated with deglutition, the vagus.
The rich connections between this 'slave nerve' and the 'choice centres' of the
brain will obviously necessitate a hierarchy of organization. With particular
reference to chewing and swallowing this hierarchy consists simply and essentially of three levels: the brain stem centres (cranial nerves, nuclei, and reticular formation), drive centres of the hypothalamus and associated structures,
and the analytical experiential centres (e.g. cerebral cortex and cerebellum)
responsible for choice or specificity and refinement of action. These three
centres find an interesting parallel in the primitive neural outgrowths of the
buccal lobe of the octopus brain (Young, 1968).

Stimulation of the appropriate region of any of the above three centres
will, irrespective of peripheral feedback, evoke recognizable chewing and swallowing patterns in the motor nerves supplying the muscles involved. But the
brain stem centres contain all the neural components essential for automatic
chewing, swallowing, and even vocalization (Bazett and Penfield, 1922). From
recent studies it appears that the brain stem contains a neural switch for
chewing that can be operated by neurotransmitters like adrenalin and seroto-
nin (Thomas, 1971). I believe it is only a matter of time before chewing and
swallowing will be produced in low-decerebrate preparations by the administration of autonomic neurotransmitters or mimetics, as has been already
demonstrated for walking in spinal and mesencephalic cats (Forssberg and
Grillner, 1973; Grillner and Shik, 1973).

Taylor and Davey (1968) in the cat, Matsunami and Kubota (1972) in the
monkey, and Peyton (1972), from my laboratory, in the rat have indicated
that the patterned output from the brain stem during chewing consists of
alpha-gamma coactivation of jaw-elevator extrafusal and spindle intrafusal

muscles respectively. Furthermore Grillner (1969) has provided convincing evidence that both static and dynamic gamma innervation of cat intrafusal fibres are under adrenergic and serotoninergic control. The licking, swallowing, sucking, and chewing automations of DOPA-treated Parkinson patients further suggests reticular formation control of these oral functions in man.

Evolution and maturation of brain activity does not depend solely upon the development of facilitatory mechanisms. Inhibition of older functions in particular clearly has a part to play, as the Babinski response strikingly exemplifies. I see Dr Storey's researches on the apnoeic response of new-born lambs to laryngeal stimulation as an even more exciting example because, apart from its fundamental importance to the understanding of brain organization in oropharyngo-laryngeal interactions, it offers an explanation for the mystifying sudden infant death syndrome which is the greatest single cause of death between one-week and one-year of age in Canada and the USA. Physiological saline might not be a sufficient chemical stimulant for obvious reasons, whereas water, as a diluent of normal secretions, could be an adequate chemical and pressure stimulus. Dawes and Mott (1959) also demonstrated that the Hering-Breuer reflex was present in the immature new-born rabbit. In this context the observation made during Storey's discussion that the inhalation of amniotic fluid in the foetus may be the adequate stimulus for respiratory inhibition is interesting. Frankstein (1970) explained the loss of the inhibitory Hering-Breuer reflex in man as being mediated by a mechanism which is always present in man but only under special circumstances in animals. I suspect the lesson we have learned from this session is that we are still working at a very superficial and speculative level in the field of swallowing and mastication and that research into the detailed mechanisms of control promises to be very productive as well as exciting.

REFERENCES

Bazett, H.C., and Penfield, W.G. 1922. A study of the Sherrington decerebrate animal in the chronic as well as the acute condition. *Brain* 45: 185–265

Dawes, G.S., and Mott, J.C. 1959. Reflex respiratory activity in the new-born rabbit. *J. Physiol. (Lond.)* 145: 85–97

Eccles, J.C. 1973. Brain, speech and consciousness. *Naturwissenschaften* 60: 167–76

Forssberg, H., and Grillner, S. 1973. The locomotion of the spinal cat injected with clonidine i.v. *Brain Res.* 50: 184–6

Frankstein, S.I. 1970. Neural control of respiration. In R. Porter (ed.),
    Breathing: Hering-Breuer Centenary Symposium. London: Churchill
Grillner, S. 1969. The influence of DOPA on the static and the dynamic fusi-
    motor activity of the triceps surae of the spinal cat. *Acta physiol. scand.*
    77: 490-509
Grillner, S., and Shik, M.L. 1973. On the descending control of the lumbo-
    sacral spinal cord from the mesencephalic locomotor region. *Acta physiol.
    scand.* 87: 320-33
Matsunami, K., and Kubota, K. 1972. Muscle afferents of trigeminal mesen-
    cephalic tract nucleus and mastication in chronic monkeys. *Jap. J. Physiol.*
    22: 545-55
Peyton, S. 1972. *Mastication in the Freely Moving Cat.* PHD Thesis, Univ. of
    Alberta
Smith, H.W. 1953. *From Fish to Philosopher.* Boston: Little, Brown
Sperry, R.W. 1968. Hemisphere deconnection and unity in conscious
    awareness. *Am. Psychol.* 23: 723-33
Taylor, A., and Davey, M.R. 1968. Behaviour of jaw muscle stretch receptors
    during active and passive movements in the cat. *Nature* 220: 301-2
Thomas, N.R. 1969. Reflex mastication and its central control in the decere-
    brate rat. *J. Canad. dent. Assoc.* 35: 273
— 1971. Neural switching device for mastication control. *Proc. 50th Gen.
    Session IADR,* p. 279, Abstract 926
Woods, R. 1964. Behavior of chronic decerebrate rats. *J. Neurophysiol.* 27:
    635-44
Young, J.Z. 1968. Influence of the mouth on the evolution of the brain.
    In P. Person (ed.), *Biology of the Mouth.* Washington: AAAS.

SECTION TWO

Mastication and swallowing:
Motoneurone mechanisms

Chairman's Introduction

B.J. SESSLE

I believe that the following questions are basic to the topic of this session. (1) What do we presently know of the reflex and central controls of oral-facial motoneurone function, what do we still need to know, and how should we attempt to provide this information? (2) How do these mechanisms compare with those operative at the spinal cord level? (3) How do these mechanisms contribute to mastication and swallowing?

The last question is probably the most important for us to consider, and there are many related questions that we must ask ourselves. Once the motoneurones involved in mastication and swallowing have been identified, can we explain the synergistic and antagonistic patterns of their activity that must occur for mastication and swallowing to be achieved? Since most of these motoneurones are active in mastication and swallowing, what gives them the green light for one activity, the red light for the other? Is it the sensory information that comes relatively direct from the periphery, or are local brain stem regions or perhaps even higher centres more important? Does sensory input in fact significantly modify their behaviour during mastication and swallowing, or are these patterns of activity intrinsic, with little chance of modification through learning? Since the motoneurones serve a protective function in addition to alimentary and respiratory ones, do the reflex and suprasegmental controls to be considered by Drs Goldberg and Kubota simply represent an overlay which takes precedence over mastication and swallowing to afford protection for oral-facial structures?

Many of these questions are probably more applicable to later sessions in this symposium and especially the first workshop report. Nevertheless, I think that they need to be asked now to give us some perspective of the topic of this present section and its relevance to mastication and swallowing.

As a starting point, let us consider the motoneurones involved in mastication and swallowing. The motoneurones that receive these reflex and higher centre inputs and that are active in mastication and swallowing lie in pools or

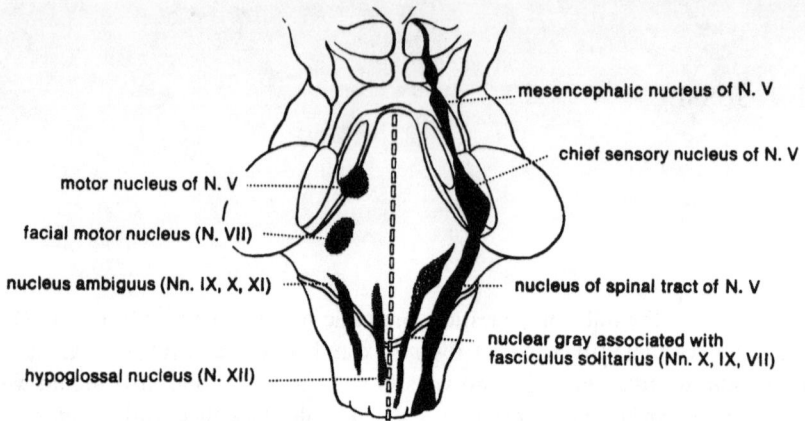

FIGURE 1 Sensory and motor nuclei of the brain stem involved in mastication and swallowing. For convenience, the sensory nuclei are shown only on the right, the motor nuclei only on the left. The nuclei are associated with cranial nerves (Nn.)V, VII, IX, X, XI, and XII.

nuclei in the pons and medulla and upper cervical spinal cord (Fig. 1). Note the close proximity to these motoneurone pools of the brain stem sensory nuclei, in particular the trigeminal and solitary tract nuclear complexes. A number of studies, both anatomical and physiological, have described direct and indirect connections between these sensory nuclei and many of these motoneurones (e.g. see papers by Goldberg; Gobel; Greenwood and Sessle, this volume). In other words, many of the interneurones involved in the transfer of incoming sensory information from the oral-facial region to these motoneurones are located in these sensory nuclei. In the past many of us have had the tendency to think of these sensory nuclei purely in terms of their relay to higher centres and their involvement in the central neural processes of perception of tactile, thermal, and noxious stimuli applied to face and mouth. But these sensory nuclei are an integral part of reflex function, and I am sure Dr Goldberg, Dr Gobel, and others will document the physiological and anatomical evidence in support of this view.

I should also point out that these motoneurones, and also the sensory neurones, receive a considerable input from higher centres as well as from the periphery. Again these descending inputs may be direct or indirect. For example, with respect to the sensorimotor cortex, there is evidence of rapidly conducting feedback loops between brain stem and cortex. Thus the motoneurones can be modulated directly or indirectly by the higher centre control of incoming sensory information, and Dr Kubota will expand on the significance of such inputs.

The mechanisms that contribute to the reflex and suprasegmental controls of these oral-facial motoneurones have only recently been studied to any great extent. In comparison, countless pages and symposia have been concerned with the spinal mechanisms contributing to posture and locomotion. But even recent works on the topics of posture and motility have largely neglected the knowledge obtained in the last 10 years of the motoneurone mechanisms contributing to oral-facial posture and movements. And many physiologists and clinicians still tend to think that these movements have a basis similar to that existing at the spinal cord. But important differences do exist, and to allow us to make comparison, I want to conclude this introduction by reviewing briefly the basic and relevant spinal mechanisms.

The limb and trunk muscles contain length-sensitive receptors, the typical one being the muscle spindle. The spindle's Ia afferent monosynaptic connection to the alpha spinal motoneurone was established by physiological studies more than 30 years ago. However, from earlier studies by Sherrington and his contemporaries, it was well known that other peripheral inputs of both muscle and cutaneous origin projected to and profoundly modified the activity of the spinal motoneurone. Sherrington's classical studies in the decerebrate and spinalized cat had established, for example, that cutaneous stimulation evokes a set pattern of postural modification. And he later suggested the spinal motoneuronal mechanisms contributing to such reflex actions. Other workers also emphasized the importance of muscle receptors in not only exciting muscles but also in depressing their activity, e.g. Golgi tendon organs and the concept of autogenic inhibition.

Such findings of both excitatory and inhibitory effects of muscle and cutaneous inputs laid the foundation for the concept of reciprocal innervation. For example, muscle spindle input from a limb extensor muscle was viewed as excitatory to the muscle and its synergists, but inhibitory to the muscle's antagonists (flexors). Moreover, the production of limb flexion by a cutaneous noxious stimulus is also achieved through reciprocal innervation – excitation of ipsilateral flexors, inhibition of ipsilateral extensors. The contralateral muscles tend to show opposite effects (double reciprocal innervation). The motoneurones, of course, also receive supraspinal inputs, and these too often have reciprocal effects on extensors and flexors.

With the advent of single-cell recording capabilities, physiologists utilized appropriate physiological and pharmacological approaches to gain some insight into the motoneuronal events that underlie these various excitatory and inhibitory influences. For example, they verified that inhibition might result from an intracellular hyperpolarization: so-called postsynaptic inhibition, but also implicated a presynaptic mechanism in some of the inhibitory influences. This 'presynaptic inhibition' is thought to be the result of a presynaptic depolarization of the sensory input to the motoneurone. Although this presynaptic inhibition might occur at the synapses on the motoneurone, in many cases it seems to have its action indirectly, by acting on the interneurones in the dorsal horn for example. A considerable amount of study has been devoted to such apparent presynaptic influences which are quite widespread within the spinal motor system and elsewhere in the brain, but the real significance of this presynaptic mechanism is still uncertain.

The single neurone studies also confirmed the existence of a gamma system in the limb muscles. Gamma motoneurones in the spinal cord receive no monosynaptic muscle spindle input but, by virtue of their efferent innervation of the spindle, can modify muscle spindle afferent discharge. Thus they can change the gain of the alpha motoneurone system and thereby influence posture and movement. As with the alpha motoneurone, suprasegmental as well as peripheral inputs project to the gamma motoneurones.

Typically then the spinal motoneurone has muscle spindle afferent input from both agonist and antagonist muscles, from other muscle afferents (e.g. Golgi tendon organs) and from cutaneous sources. Reciprocal influences from the periphery are also accompanied by reciprocal effects of higher centres and these inputs have been thought to provide the basis for posture and coordinated movement. Inherent in such a view are the underlying contributions of the gamma system, postsynaptic and presynaptic inhibition, etc. Let us now consider whether similar afferent systems and mechanisms operate at the brain stem level to contribute to the motility patterns required for mastication and swallowing and associated oral-facial movements.

Motoneurone mechanisms: reflex controls

L.J. GOLDBERG

This is a rather broad area in which a large body of literature has developed in recent years. I shall attempt, however, to maintain a fairly wide focus in order to give some attention to many of the various approaches which exist in the study of the reflex control of mastication and swallowing. Although it would be possible to consider separately the major motoneurone groups directly involved in these two functions (i.e., trigeminal, facial, glossopharyngeal, vagal, and hypoglossal) and to discuss the great variety of reflexes with which they are involved, it is more appropriate and, I hope, will prove to be more interesting to consider these motoneurones and the peripheral influences that affect them in the context of their participation in the acts of mastication and swallowing.

The chew and the swallow can be considered from the two opposite poles of the universe. At one pole, the one located furthest from reality, is the neurophysiological preparation, and at the other is the ceaselessly chewing and swallowing human being who has the understandable desire to maintain his chewing and swallowing apparatus in excellent operating condition. Since my own grasp of the latter reality has its shortcomings, I am going to view mastication and swallowing from the perspective of the neurophysiological preparation.

The neurophysiologist attempts to isolate and study the various elements that participate in a particular activity. In doing so, the neurophysiologist moves, comfortably or distressingly depending on one's point of view, away from the totality of the act he attempts to understand. Accepting this constraint for a moment, let us examine the view of mastication and swallowing one gets from the neurophysiological perspective.

SWALLOWING

It has been well established in animal preparations that swallowing can be triggered by appropriate stimuli from the periphery (Doty and Bosma, 1956;

Storey, 1968; Miller and Loizzi, 1974). The interesting feature of the swallowing induced in the animal preparation is that, once the peripheral stimulus has successfully initiated the beginning of a swallow, there occurs a precisely ordered march of activity of muscles innervated by motoneurones whose axons travel in the vth, viith, ixth, xth and xiith cranial nerves (Doty and Bosma, 1956). Once begun, this stereotyped pattern of response is consistently repeated from one swallow to the next. The pattern remains consistent even without the benefit of sensory feedback to the brain stem (Sumi, 1970a; Miller, 1972a). The necessary element for the coordinated activity of the motoneurones involved is the 'swallowing centre' which has been located in the medullary reticular formation (Doty, Richmond, and Storey, 1967; Miller, 1972b; Sumi, 1972).

We have, therefore, a model of swallowing which suggests that appropriate peripheral activity can trigger reticular formation neurones in the 'swallowing centre'; this triggered 'swallowing centre' has the capability to command sequentially the appropriate motoneurones in order to produce a swallow. I am not aware of any studies that indicate how the 'swallowing centre' works this magic. However, it is only in invertebrate systems that neurophysiologists have been able to study in depth similar types of command centres and the resulting complex behaviours they control.

The above discussion would indicate that the only effect peripheral input has on swallowing is the ability to trigger it. This is not the case. Peripheral influences do appear to have an important, if indirect, effect on swallowing. It has been reported that a continuous train of electrical shocks delivered to the lingual nerve of anaesthetized cats blocks swallowing induced by superior laryngeal nerve stimulation, as well as inhibiting the bursting activity of hypoglossal motoneurones associated with each swallow (Sumi, 1970b). This inhibition of hypoglossal motoneurone activity continued to be present when the animal was paralyzed. In addition, evidence has recently been presented which suggests that activity from the periphery may determine when a swallow can occur by modulating the effectiveness of the triggering input to activate the 'swallowing centre' (Sessle and Storey, 1972; Sessle, 1973a,b). It has been shown that electrical stimulation of the infraorbital, superior laryngeal, and glossopharyngeal nerves, or mechanical stimulation of the maxillary canine and upper lip, produces presynaptic depolarization in the central terminals of the superior laryngeal nerve which are located in the nucleus of the solitary tract (Sessle, 1973b). These afferent fibres presumably include those which mediate triggering of the 'swallowing centre' when the laryngeal mucosa is stimulated or when electric shocks are delivered to the superior laryngeal nerve itself. Furthermore, the activation of neurones in the nucleus of the solitary tract by superior laryngeal nerve stimulation could be suppressed by conditioning stimuli delivered to the superior laryngeal and glossopharyn-geal nerves. Conditioning stimuli delivered to the infraorbital nerve or maxil-lary canine tooth were also found to be effective (Sessle, 1973a).

The hypothesis has been stated that the periodontal receptor stimulation which occurs during chewing might be important in determining when a swal-low will occur by affecting the level of polarization in the terminals of those afferents mediating the triggering input. If the level of depolarization was suf-ficiently elevated, then swallowing would not occur, having become the victim of presynaptic inhibition (Sessle and Storey, 1972). The possibility exists, therefore, that if the food bolus is tough there will be a great deal of perio-dontal receptor activity and a concurrent inhibition of the onset of swallow-ing. If the food bolus were of a soft consistency and minimally activated periodontal receptors, then swallowing would not be impeded and could occur after only a few chewing movements.

Another neurophysiological demonstration of possible mastication-swal-lowing interaction is the finding that there are neurones in the reticular for-mation adjacent to the solitary tract which can be driven by superior laryngeal and glossopharyngeal nerve stimulation; and that 40 per cent of these neu-rones project rostrally to the vicinity of the trigeminal motor nucleus. The possibility here is that these reticular formation neurones are involved in some form of coordination of swallowing and mastication (Sessle, 1973a).

MASTICATION

The ability of peripheral stimuli to induce swallowing leads one to the ques-tion: can stimulation from the periphery trigger mastication?The answer is clearly, 'maybe.' Rhythmic chewing movements in lightly anaesthetized and decerebrate rabbits have been elicited when a balloon was placed at the back of the mouth (Lund and Dellow, 1971). In the encéphale isolé cat, rhythmic bursts of activity corresponding to jaw-opening movements were recorded from the digastric nerve (Denavit-Saubié and Corvisier, 1972). This bursting activity, while occurring spontaneously, was reported to be more frequently observed when an object was placed in the animal's mouth and could persist for 5 to 30 minutes. The authors also state that the rhythmicity could be re-triggered by tactile stimulation at the corners of the mouth or by slight movement of the object in the mouth. Sixty-two of one hundred and eighty interneurones recorded from throughout the trigeminal motor nucleus de-monstrated rhythmic firing patterns which were related to the digastric nerve discharges. The hypothesis was put forth that these interneurones are impli-cated in the generation of rhythmic masticatory movements (Denavit-Saubié and Corvisier, 1972). It has also been reported that a constant diffuse application of force applied to the palate of decerebrate cats can elicit rhythmic bursts of activity in digastric and intrinsic tongue muscles. No such activity was recorded from the jaw-closing temporalis muscle. The burst duration was 100–150 msec and occurred 4–5 times a second. The digastric and tongue muscle activities had the same periodicity but were not in phase with each other. Rhythmic bursts of activity recorded in the cut hypoglossal nerve evoked by a diffuse stimulus to the palate was reported to persist, apparently unchanged, after paralysis of the animal (Thexton, 1973).

It appears from these studies that peripheral input can elicit rhythmic activity in trigeminal and hypoglossal motoneurones. The relationship of this rhythmic activity to the behaviour we call mastication is, however, far more tenuous than the swallowing that could be triggered by superior laryngeal nerve stimulation.

Stimulation of suprasegmental systems has been shown to lead to rhythmic chewing movements and these will be discussed by Dr Kubota. I shall only make two brief points concerning the relationship of segmental influences to this phenomenon: (1) suprasegmentally evoked chewing movements are independent of feedback from the periphery; (2) they strongly interact with feedback from the periphery. In support of the first point is a study in which suprasegmentally evoked alternating discharges in nerves to jaw-opening and jaw-closing muscles were not affected by paralysis (Dellow and Lund, 1971). With regard to the second point, segmental input clearly has been shown to interact with suprasegmentally evoked rhythmic activity (Lund and Dellow, 1971; Morimoto and Kawamura, 1973). Further discussion on the relationship of sensory feedback to suprasegmentally evoked chewing activity will be undertaken later in this book.

Although rhythmic activity in motoneurones involved in chewing may be controlled to some extent by a brain stem 'chewing centre,' there is no doubt that receptors in many parts of the oral-pharyngeal area have direct and powerful lines of communication to these motoneurones. A great number of reflexes have been described involving motoneurones of the trigeminal, facial, and hypoglossal nerves. The study of these reflexes usually entails delivering an electrical shock to a sensory nerve while observing the effects of the stimulation on interneurones and motoneurones in the brain stem, or on the masticatory muscles themselves. More natural stimuli such as a controlled pressure to a tooth or the stretch of a muscle have also been employed. A list of the peripheral influences (excluding pain) which are known to have a reflex effect on the previously mentioned major motoneurone groups involved in chewing would include: temporomandibular joint mechanoreceptors; intra-oral mucosa mechanoreceptors, including those of the tongue, gingiva, periodontal

ligaments, and palate; pharyngeal and laryngeal mucosal receptors; mechanoreceptors in the lips and skin of the face; muscle proprioceptors in the masticatory and facial muscles, as well as specialized receptors in the tongue. There
is a growing number of papers on all these topics and a review in this area has
recently been published (Kawamura, 1974).

It would be impossible, and not particularly useful, to summarize these
studies at this point. Instead, I should like to discuss recent neurophysiological experiments in the cat which have forced a reassessment of the classic theory concerning reflex control of mastication first proposed by Sherrington
(1917), and more recently modified by Jerge (1964). The original hypothesis
described the cyclic nature of chewing as originating from the interaction
between two oral reflexes. One aspect of the hypothesis was based on the
observation that mechanical stimulation of intra-oral receptors or electrical
stimulation of their afferent nerves resulted in jaw opening via excitation of
jaw-depressor muscles such as the digastric, accompanied by inhibition of jaw
elevators. Recent studies, however, have demonstrated that electrical stimulation of low-threshold afferent fibres supplying the oral mucosa result in a
much more complex series of events than jaw-opening motoneurone excitation and jaw-closer inhibition.

A single shock stimulus to low-threshold afferents in the lingual or inferior
dental nerve results in at least two distinct inhibitory processes in motoneurones of the masseter muscles (Goldberg and Nakamura, 1968; Kidokoro
et al., 1968a). The first phase is an inhibitory postsynaptic potential (IPSP)
with a latency of approximately 2 msec and a duration of approximately 15
msec. The second phase peaks at a latency of about 40 msec and can continue
for 100–400 msec. There is evidence that the two phases are distinct in terms
of mechanism of action and neuronal pathway. The first phase involves activation of interneurones in the supratrigeminal nucleus (Goldberg and Nakamura,
1968; Kidokoro et al., 1968b). In studies using the monosynaptic masseteric
reflex as a test of masseter motoneurone excitability, it was found that the
second phase is dependent upon a path which descends caudal to the trigeminal motor nucleus since lesions of the brain stem approximately 3 mm below
the motor nucleus abolished the second phase without affecting the first
(Goldberg and Nakamura, 1968; Sumino, 1971).

To complicate matters a bit more it was discovered that intra-oral nerve
stimulation also activated a reflex excitatory to jaw-closing motoneurones
(Goldberg, 1971, 1972a,b; Sumino, 1971; Sessle and Schmitt, 1972). This
excitatory influence had not been previously observed because it was masked
by the inhibitory effects.

So we are faced with a situation in which stimulation of low-threshold
afferents in nerves supplying the mucosa of the mouth does not merely inhi-

bit jaw-closing motoneurones as required by the hypothesis but results in two types of inhibitory effects and a simultaneous excitatory effect.

Pleasantly enough for the hypothesis, stimulation of these intra-oral afferent nerves does evoke a simple excitation of digastric motoneurones, and the excitation occurs during the first phase of jaw-closer motoneurone inhibition. There remains, however, one further complication to the story. The ability of a volley of impulses in large afferent fibres in the inferior dental or lingual nerve to either excite digastric motoneurones or inhibit masseteric motoneurones can be reduced by prior activity in these same nerves on the contralateral side (Goldberg, 1972b; Goldberg and Browne, 1974). This inhibition of reflex activity by the conditioning input has been postulated as due to depolarization of the terminals of the primary afferent fibres mediating the test reflex. These findings lead to the conclusion that the reflexes have been inhibited presynaptically (Goldberg, 1972b; Goldberg and Browne, 1974).

Unfortunately, little can be said at present about the function, if any, of presynaptic inhibition in motor control (Granit, 1970; Burke, 1971; Schmidt, 1971). A proposed role for presynaptic inhibition in the initiation of swallowing has already been discussed. An attempt has been made to determine if there is some pattern of organization for presynaptic inhibition with respect to reflexes involved in mastication (Goldberg and Browne, 1974). The excitability of the digastric reflex when evoked by the ipsilateral lingual or inferior dental nerve was tested following a conditioning stimulus to either of the same nerves on the contralateral side. The conditioning stimulus was adjusted so as to be subthreshold for evoking a digastric reflex on the test side. Beginning after a latency of approximately 15-20 msec, the test reflex was inhibited by the conditioning stimulus. A difference in time course of this inhibition was observed which was not dependent on the site of the conditioning stimulus, but rather on whether the test reflex was evoked by the ipsilateral lingual or inferior dental nerve. A similar difference in time course was found for the increase in excitability of lingual as compared to inferior dental nerve terminals in the trigeminal main sensory nucleus to conditioning stimuli delivered to either of the contralateral nerves (Goldberg and Browne, 1974). Here we have, then, a case in which two similar oral reflexes could be distinguished by the character of their response to intra-oral peripheral influences which evoke primary afferent depolarization. There is, therefore, at least some differentiation in the effect of primary afferent depolarization on trigeminal reflexes.

To this complex array of reflex effects we must add the work of Nakamura and his group who have described presynaptic inhibition of the digastric reflex resulting from stimulation of high-threshold afferents in the nerve to the masseter muscle (Nakamura and Wu, 1970). They have also recently begun to identify the contribution of these muscle afferents to reflexes of both ipsilateral and contralateral jaw elevator and depressor motoneurones (Nakamura et al., 1973a,b).

CONCLUSION

We have immersed ourselves in the cozy world of the neurophysiological preparation. As can be seen there is quite enough in that world to keep us busy and I have not discussed the areas of tongue-jaw reflex interaction and temporomandibular joint receptor reflexes, both because of lack of space and because of the limited amount of information available at present concerning the latter. Also missing is consideration of reflexes involving the lateral pterygoid muscle since there is very little data to consider. This is a gap of immense proportions in our attempt to understand reflex controls in mastication. To a large extent the blame for this rests with the cats, our favourite neurophysiological preparation, and their consistent disinterest in lateral jaw movements. In the more cooperative rabbit a lateral jaw-movement reflex has been described (Lund, McLachlan, and Dellow, 1971).

In swallowing, the reticular formation stands between the periphery and participating motoneurones. In mastication, the motoneurones are not so protected and are bombarded by a mass of sensory feedback which, in one case, can exert its influence monosynaptically, and in others directly through interneurones in the neighbouring trigeminal sensory nucleus.

Time begins, in most reflex studies, with the onset of the stimulus. This is useful in the study of swallowing which itself can be thought of as a complex reflex. It is less successful in helping us understand mastication. Mastication is not a reflex and cannot be confined within the framework of a rigidly fixed pattern of response to an appropriate stimulus. There may be a central timing mechanism for chewing movements, and well-defined reflexes which obligate muscle groups to act in certain coordinated patterns. However, mastication must eventually be understood in the context of a continuous process of interaction between sensory feedback influences and commands from central control systems; further consideration of these points is given in the first workshop report.

Reflex studies serve the purpose of identifying the components of the segmental systems and describing their characteristics. This is not an insignificant task since these reflexes are as much a part of the substructure of the behaviours that we are interested in understanding as is the anatomy of the bones and muscles themselves.

REFERENCES

Burke, R.E. 1971. Control systems operating on spinal reflex mechanisms. *Neurosci. Res. Prog. Bull.* 9: 60–85

Dellow, P.G., and Lund, J.P. 1971. Evidence for central timing of rhythmical mastication. *J. Physiol. (Lond.)* 215: 1–13

Denavit-Saubié, M., and Corvisier, J. 1972. Cat trigeminal motor nucleus: rhythmic units firing in relation to opening movements of the mouth. *Brain Res.* 40: 500–3

Doty, R.W., and Bosma, J.F. 1956. An electromyographic analysis of reflex deglutition. *J. Neurophysiol.* 19: 61–74

Doty, R.W., Richmond, W.H., and Storey, A.T. 1967. Effect of medullary lesions on coordination of deglutition. *Exp. Neurol.* 17: 91–106

Goldberg, L.J. 1971. Masseter muscle excitation induced by stimulation of periodontal and gingival receptors in man. *Brain Res.* 32: 369–81

— 1972a. An excitatory component of the jaw opening reflex in the temporal and masseter muscles of cats and monkeys. *Experientia* 28: 44–6

— 1972b. Excitatory and inhibitory effects of lingual nerve stimulation on reflexes controlling the activity of masseteric motoneurones. *Brain Res.* 39: 95–108

Goldberg, L.J., and Browne, P.A. 1974. Differences in the excitability of two populations of trigeminal primary afferent terminals. *Brain Res.* 77: 195–209

Goldberg, L.J., and Nakamura, Y. 1968. Lingually induced inhibition of masseteric motoneurones. *Experientia* 24: 371–3

Granit, R. 1970. *The Basis of Motor Control.* London: Academic Press

Jerge, C.R. 1964. The neurologic mechanism underlying cyclic jaw movements. *J. prosth. Dent.* 14: 667–81

Kawamura, Y. 1974. Neurogenesis of mastication. In Y. Kawamura (ed.), *Frontiers of Oral Physiology.* Vol. 1. *Physiology of Mastication.* Basel: Karger

Kidokoro, Y., Kubota, K., Shuto, S., and Sumino, R. 1968a. Reflex organization of cat masticatory muscles. *J. Neurophysiol.* 31: 695–708

— 1968b. Possible interneurons responsible for reflex inhibition of motoneurons of jaw-closing muscles from the inferior dental nerve. *J. Neurophysiol.* 31: 709–16

Lund, J.P., and Dellow, P.G. 1971. The influence of interactive stimuli on rhythmical masticatory movements in rabbits. *Archs oral Biol.* 16: 215–23

Lund, J.P., McLachlan, R.S., and Dellow, P.G. 1971. A lateral jaw movement reflex. *Exp. Neurol.* 31: 189–99

Miller, A.J. 1972a. Significance of sensory inflow to the swallowing reflex. *Brain. Res.* 43: 147–59

— 1972b. Characteristics of the swallowing reflex induced by peripheral nerve and brain stem stimulation. *Exp. Neurol.* 34: 210-22

Miller, A.J., and Loizzi, R.F. 1974. Anatomical and functional differentiation of superior laryngeal nerve fibers affecting swallowing and respiration. *Exp. Neurol.* 42: 369–87

Morimoto, T., and Kawamura, Y. 1973. Properties of tongue and jaw movements elicited by stimulation of the orbital gyrus in the cat. *Archs oral Biol.* 18: 361–72

Nakamura, Y., and Wu, C.Y. 1970. Presynaptic inhibition of jaw-opening reflex by high threshold afferents from the masseter muscle of the cat. *Brain Res.* 23: 193–211

Nakamura, Y., Nagashima, H., and Mori, S. 1973a. Bilateral effects of the afferent impulses from the masseteric muscle on the trigeminal motoneuron of the cat. *Brain Res.* 57: 15–27

Nakamura, Y., Mori, S., and Nagashima, H. 1973b. Origin and central pathways of crossed inhibitory effects of afferents from the masseteric muscle on the masseteric motoneuron of the cat. *Brain Res.* 57: 29–42

Schmidt, R.F. 1971. Presynaptic inhibition in the vertebrate central nervous system. *Ergeb. Physiol.* 63: 20–101

Sessle, B.J. 1973a. Excitatory and inhibitory inputs to single neurones in the solitary tract nucleus and adjacent reticular formation. *Brain Res.* 53: 319–31

— 1973b. Presynaptic excitability changes induced in single laryngeal primary afferent fibres. *Brain Res.* 53: 333–42

Sessle, B.J., and Schmitt, A. 1972. Effects of controlled tooth stimulation on jaw muscle activity in man. *Archs oral Biol.* 17: 1597-607

Sessle, B.J., and Storey, A.T. 1972. Periodontal and facial influences on the laryngeal input to the brain stem of the cat. *Archs oral Biol.* 17: 1583–95

Sherrington, C.S. 1917. Reflexes elicitable in the cat from pinna, vibrissae and jaws. *J. Physiol. (Lond.)* 51: 404–31

Storey, A.T. 1968. Laryngeal initiation of swallowing. *Exp. Neurol.* 20: 359–65

Sumi, T. 1970a. Activity in single hypoglossal fibers during cortically induced swallowing and chewing in rabbits. *Pflügers Arch.* 314: 329–46

— 1970b. Changes of hypoglossal nerve activity during inhibition of chewing and swallowing by lingual nerve stimulation. *Pflügers Arch.* 317: 303–9

— 1972. Role of the pontine reticular formation in the neural organization of deglutition. *Jap. J. Physiol.* 22: 295–314

Sumino, R. 1971. Central neural pathways involved in the jaw-opening reflex
    in the cat. In R. Dubner and Y. Kawamura (eds.), *Oral-Facial Sensory and
    Motor Mechanisms.* New York: Appleton-Century-Crofts
Thexton, A.J. 1973. Oral reflexes elicited by mechanical stimulation of
    palatal mucosa in the cat. *Archs oral Biol.* 18: 971–80

DISCUSSION

LUND   How generalized is this inhibitory-excitatory-inhibitory pattern? Is it
true for spinal levels as well? It may also occur in the cortex and thalamus
(B.J. Sessle and R. Dubner, *Exp. Neurol.* 30 [1971]: 239–50; J.P. Lund and
B.J. Sessle, *Exp. Neurol.* 45 [1974]: 314–31).

GOLDBERG   I do not think you would find this sort of pattern in the spinal
cord. The anatomy is different and the organization of the sensory system in
relation to the motor system is different.

SESSLE   The type and function of muscle fibres innervated by the motoneurone might be an important consideration. Cutaneous afferents can produce
excitatory and/or inhibitory effects on spinal motoneurones, the dominating
effect being dependent on the property of the muscle fibres as well as the intensity of the cutaneous stimulus (e.g. R. Burke et al., *Proc. Soc. Neurosci.*
45.5 [1973]).

MATTHEWS   It is interesting to note that Sherrington actually described the
conversion of a jaw-opening reflex elicited by electrical stimulation to a jaw-
closing reflex after intravenous tetanus toxin and strychnine (C.S. Sherrington, *The Integrative Action of the Nervous System* [New Haven: Yale Univ.
Press, 1906]).

GOLDBERG   If one is focusing on the cutaneous or mucosal mechanoreceptors and stimulating only the large afferent fibres, then the motoneurone presumably gets three different kinds of messages, one inhibitory, one excitatory
and another inhibitory. One wonders what kind of message the motoneurone
receives from the receptors in the normal functional state.

DUBNER   Maybe we do have some evidence of what happens under more natural circumstances. It depends upon the situation. For example, as Thexton
(1973) has shown, jaw position to a large extent influences the sort of reflex
response one is likely to see. I think we have to get away from our simple reflex
models in order to understand what is taking place in the functional animal.

SESSLE   Thexton's work also shows that the manner in which the reflexes
behave depends upon the way the stimuli are presented. For example, if the
mechanical stimulus is prolonged (e.g. rubbing the palate) it evokes a response
with different characteristics to one evoked by a transient tactile stimulus.

GOLDBERG   The classical reflex studies do, however, give you some clue as to what the general framework is.

MATTHEWS   Are we absolutely convinced that there is a jaw-closing reflex in these situations? It is something we have to be absolutely certain about. If there is a positive feedback system from the teeth and mucous membranes to the jaw-closing muscles, then this is a very strange system. One can visualize the inhibitory pathways as providing important control in normal function, but it does seem improbable that a positive feedback system could operate without ever breaking away to cause powerful spasm of the elevator muscles (B. Matthews, in C. Lavelle (ed.), *The Applied Physiology of the Mouth* [Bristol: Wright, 1975]).

GOLDBERG   I think one has to take the view that there is a jaw-closing reflex. One sees it in neurophysiological experiments.

MATTHEWS   Maybe, but the evidence is not always straightforward. Take for example the experiments that you cite (e.g. Sumino, 1971; Goldberg, 1972b) in which effects have been observed on the monosynaptic masseteric reflex evoked by stimulation of the trigeminal mesencephalic nucleus. This stimulus does not produce a pure excitation of Ia afferents. Periodontal afferents are also being stimulated and one of the effects of this will be to bombard the periodontal fibres antidromically and block any activity passing centrally. One might also be resetting the receptors for several milliseconds.

GOLDBERG   I do believe that the excitatory influence is there. I have seen it when recording intracellularly from motoneurones responding to intraoral afferent stimulation. This forces us to reconsider the framework of the last few years. On the other hand it is possible, considering your argument about the negative effects of positive feedback, that this excitatory phenomenon may turn out not to be operant in normal chewing.

MATTHEWS   We have been looking for evidence for the existence of positive feedback in muscle control in other parts of the body. There seems to be only one mammalian situation where experimental work suggests that there may be positive feedback viz. experiments on tracking movements and the effects of anaesthesia of the skin (C.D. Marsden et al., *J. Physiol. (Lond.)* 216 [1971] : 21P). There is also evidence of a tension-based positive feedback loop in the crab (B.M.H. Bush and A.J. Cannone, *J. Physiol. (Lond.)* 236 [1974] : 37P).

SESSLE   I think the possibility of a long-loop servo involving higher centres was also mentioned.

MATTHEWS   Yes. Although there does seem to be some brain stem influence.

GREENWOOD   We have been looking at the ways in which motoneurones can be activated or facilitated, using a wide range of inputs, for example, the superior laryngeal nerve, glossopharyngeal nerve, tooth pulp, tooth tap, etc. Although we may not see all the excitation that is possible because the ani-

mals are anaesthetized or decerebrate, and although we have not used strychnine, a large proportion of digastric motoneurones receive excitatory inputs
from all these sites. In contrast, the elevator motoneurones are rarely excited
by any of these inputs except tooth tapping (see paper by Greenwood and
Sessle, this volume). Even here there is the possibility that electrotonic coupling may be occurring in the mesencephalic nucleus.

GOLDBERG   Once again, this highlights the differences that exist between the
trigeminal system and the spinal cord. We have a double pathway to the brain
stem for afferent information from the oral mucosa: one via the gasserian
ganglion and the other via the mesencephalic nucleus.

KAWAMURA   As I mentioned earlier, there are very few muscle spindles in
the depressor muscles. This also emphasizes the differences between the
spinal cord and brain stem. Recently we have been carrying out some experiments on the relationships between masseteric and digastric motoneurones
and the trigeminal caudal nucleus. Electrical stimulation of the digastric
branch produced an IPSP with a latency of 30 msec in the masseteric motoneurones. As the stimulus became stronger, the latency of the IPSP became
shorter. In the digastric motoneurones, stimulation of high-threshold caudal
fibres induced an EPSP with about 5 msec latency and it was followed by an
IPSP. Weak stimulation of the masseteric nerve at less than ten times threshold
did not produce any effects on the digastric motoneurones. Ia afferents from
the masseter nerve do not project to digastric motoneurones. It therefore
seems that the digastric motoneurone appears to be influenced by impulses
from high-threshold afferent nerve fibres of the masseter muscle, and that the
masseteric motoneurone is influenced by digastric high-threshold afferents
(Kawamura, 1974).

SESSLE   We have also found similar effects from high-threshold muscle afferents. The reciprocal relationship seen in spinal motoneurones with low-
threshold muscle afferents is apparently lacking in cranial motoneurones, although Group II jaw muscle afferent effects may fit the spinal picture (Nakamura et al., 1973a).

THOMAS   In the rat I have stimulated the palatal nerves and obtained a reflex
that has as short a latency as the masseteric monosynaptic reflex. I have
traced the neurones involved and they clearly pass up to the mesencephalic
nucleus and from there down to the motor nucleus, to the digastric motoneurones. It is a very interesting pathway, and I am hesitant to mention it because
it breaks the fundamental rule that the only monosynaptic reflex we have involves the muscle spindle.

SESSLE   Some of the latencies Dr Greenwood and I noted in masseter motoneurones with tooth tap stimulation suggest that there may be monosynaptic

connections, but we have found no evidence that there are monosynaptic connections associated with digastric motoneurones. This, of course, is in the cat, and there may be species differences.

THOMAS The species difference may be very important because the temporomandibular joint in the rodent allows anteroposterior movement, whereas that in the cat does not.

Motoneurone mechanisms: suprasegmental controls

KISOU KUBOTA

According to the traditional view of the central control of movement, structures at the lower level of the brain provide inherent reflex mechanisms while structures at higher levels supply modulating mechanisms, so that reflexes are efficiently and reasonably realized. This modulation may be accomplished by the reception of sensory information from given muscles and by the outflow of efferent influences to various neurones at the lower level. Thus, the presence of feedback loops are presupposed.

Although higher structures, such as the neocortex, limbic cortex, and hypothalamus can modulate mastication and swallowing, little is known about their physiological roles in the control of these functions and how the higher structures are influenced by various afferent inputs. My topic will concentrate on relations between the rostral part of the cerebrum and motoneurones and on unit activity in the precentral cortex.

FACE MOTOR CORTEX

Stimulation and lesion studies give only a first-order approximation of the functions of a given structure. Almost a century has passed since Ferrier (1876) found that stimulation of the lateral part of the precentral cortex evokes jaw movement, but we have still to discover the first-order estimate of effects of cortical stimulation with respect to mastication and swallowing. Lesion studies have failed to show clear deficits (Green and Walker, 1938), although it is now established in the rat, rabbit, cat, dog, monkey, and human that the dorsolateral or anterolateral part of the frontal cortex, if stimulated repetitively, induces a series of masticatory and swallowing movements (cf. Woolsey et al., 1952; Tsukamoto, 1963; Kawamura, 1964; Sumi, 1969). However, cortical representation of masticatory muscles in the precentral motor cortex is somewhat unclear and representation of muscles for swallowing has not been studied (cf. O'Brien, Pimpaneau, and Albe-Fessard, 1971) although laryngeal muscle representation has been reported (Hast et al., 1974).

While Sherrington (Leyton and Sherrington, 1917; Sherrington, 1947) clearly noted a cortical representation of jaw opening and jaw closing in cat and monkey, Woolsey's group (1952) could not induce good movements of the jaw from the precentral area in rhesus and java monkeys. Chewing is rarely induced with simultaneous facial movements, but swallowing is induced more commonly. This discrepancy seems to depend upon differences of the stimulus parameters and the level of anaesthesia used. In deeply anaesthetized monkeys, cortical surface stimulation never, or only occasionally, induces reproducible jaw movement (Walker and Green, 1938; Hines, 1940). Stimulation of a more lateral area (area 6) is capable of inducing rhythmic chewing (cf. Vogt and Vogt, 1919; Lund and Lamarre, 1974) which persists after removing area 4 (Walker and Green, 1938). Hence this part is appropriately designated as the cortical masticatory area (Lund and Lamarre, 1974). Whether in lower animals there is an anatomically and physiologically different area from the face motor cortex from which mastication and swallowing can be evoked, is yet to be determined.

If the precentral cortex is electrically excited, flexor facilitation is more easily evoked and extensor facilitation is less commonly evoked. This has been confirmed repeatedly, in a variety of animal species, by many studies of forelimb and hindlimb muscles or motoneurones. A recent study by Chase and McGinty (1970b) has shown that this is also the case for the masticatory muscles. In the unanaesthetized, immobilized squirrel monkey the reflex activity of the digastric nerve was recorded after shocks to the lingual or inferior dental nerve; the reflex activity of the masseter nerve was recorded after shocks to the mesencephalic tract nucleus. The cortical surface was stimulated by single shocks or trains of pulses, and effects upon evoked reflex activities were studied. While facilitation of the digastric reflex activity was obtained by threshold stimulation from a relatively circumscribed area, inhibition of the masseteric monosynaptic reflex occurred from a wider area of the lateral surface of the cortex. Threshold intensity was usually lower for digastric facilitation than for masseteric inhibition. It is difficult to account for the masseter inhibition only as a reciprocal inhibition associated with digastric facilitation. Two possibilities may exist: that cortical activation of muscles other than the digastric muscle, such as the tongue or laryngeal muscles, is inducing associated reciprocal inhibition of the masseter muscle, or that there is a nonreciprocal, inhibitory mechanism which suppresses the movements non-specifically. It has long been known that stimulation of the orbital gyrus is capable of inducing the state of behavioural inhibition or sleep (cf. Sauerland et al., 1967). By its stimulation, various somatomotor and visceromotor activities are depressed (Kaada, 1951; Sauerland et al., 1967). However, the stimulated area is close to the area from which facial, tongue and jaw movements can be evoked (Porter, 1967; Chase and McGinty, 1970a; Limansky, Pilyavsky and

Gura, 1971, 1972; Woody, 1974). Therefore, influences on cranial motoneurones must be carefully studied, with consideration given to the precise extent
of the effective cortical area.

Stimulation studies were further extended from the surface to depths
within the motor cortex. Clark and Luschei (1974) showed in a brief report
that jaw opening or jaw closing are produced separately or concurrently by
intracortical microstimulation of motor cortex area 4. However, the exact
stimulus locations were not detailed. It has still to be demonstrated whether
or not tongue or lip movements are simultaneously evoked by a minimal current intensity. I believe that their results will provide strong evidence for masticatory representation within the face motor cortex.

Dr H. Asanuma and I have also tried to stimulate the face motor cortex of
two Cebus monkeys by an intracortical microstimulation method, in order to
examine the effects on jaw movements. Electrodes were glass-coated tungsten
electrodes (Stoney, Thompson, and Asanuma, 1968). Surgery was performed
with the animals anaesthetized with halothane. A small dose of barbiturate
(Nembutal, 10 mg/kg) was also given initially, and later during experiments
an additional dose (5 mg/kg) was administered whenever the monkey became
unstable. Care was taken to eliminate pain. Each monkey was placed in a primate chair and the skull was fixed to the chair by bolts and dental cement.
The cortical surface was exposed and the area penetrated as illustrated in Figure 1. In total, 40 penetrations were performed. By surface monopolar catho-
dal stimulation (0.2 msec, 300 Hz for 40 msec), lip or mouth movements
could be evoked (0.7-1.5 mA) ipsilaterally or contralaterally from the dorsolateral cortex and from behind the arcuate sulcus close to the central sulcus.
However, clear jaw movements were never observed. Below the cortical surface, stimulation (4-10 μA) induced tongue retraction and extension or lateral deflection of both lower and upper lips, but visible jaw movements were
not evoked at intensities of less than 50 μA.

Figure 1 also illustrates an example of an abridged protocol of a single
penetration. At various depths the threshold intensity required to activate
various muscles is illustrated. Whether the area is represented ipsilaterally or
contralaterally was not confirmed (cf. Lauer, 1952). Jaw opening was searched
for with the animal's mouth closed, and jaw closing with its jaw open. If an
appropriate site deep in the arm motor cortex was stimulated, finger movements were evoked (Asanuma and Sakata, 1967) at an intensity of less than
5 μA. The stimulus intensity (usually 100 or 200 μA, 0.2 msec, 200 Hz, 175-
200 msec) used by Clark and Luschei for inducing jaw movements was
stronger than the cortical stimuli used in our study. This factor and the use of
light barbiturate anaesthesia by us might account for the differences in the
findings.

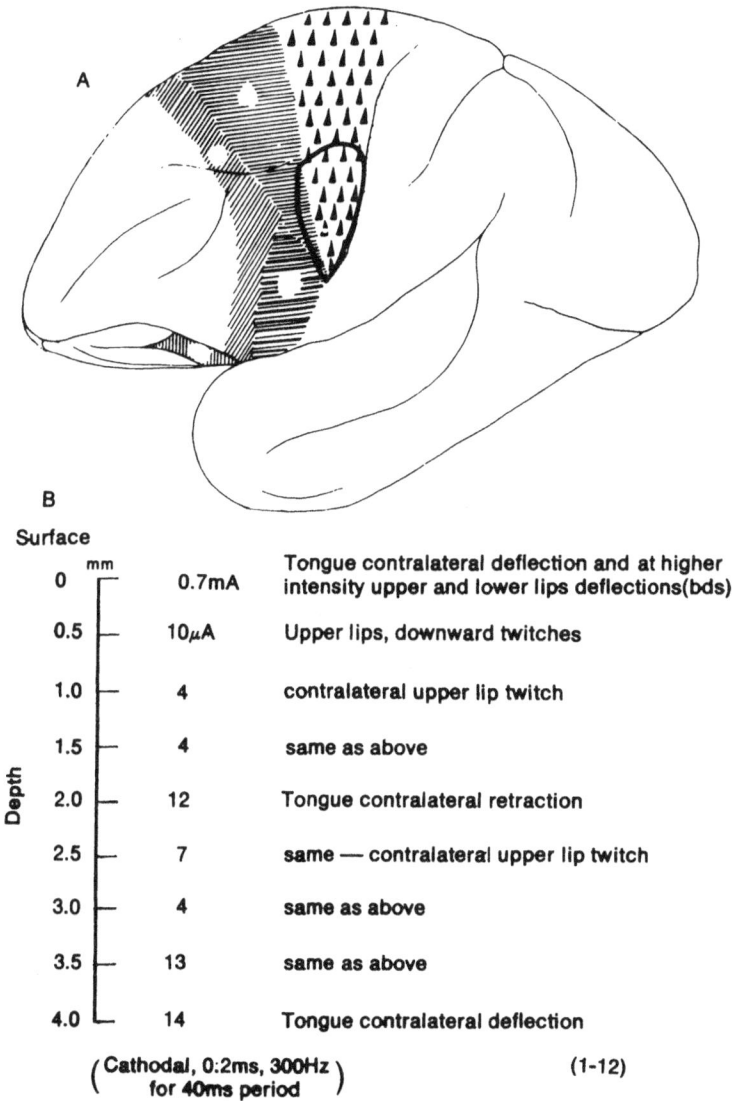

FIGURE 1 A: Lateral view of the precentral cortex of the Cebus monkey (see von Bonin, 1949). A circle at the lateral part of area 4 indicates the place where electrode penetrations for microstimulation were performed. A triangle with a blank dot in the centre, the most rostral triangle of the third line from the bottom, indicates a penetrated site from which the responses indicated in B were evoked. B: Responses during micro-stimulations at various depths in the face motor area in a Cebus monkey. Stimulus sites are indicated in A. Reproduced from *Precentral Motor Cortex*, P.C. Bucy (ed.), Urbana, Ill.: U. of Illinois Press (courtesy of the publisher and author).

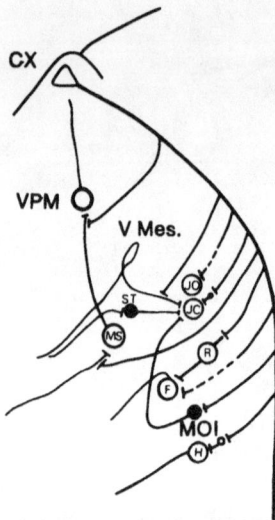

FIGURE 2 Schematic illustration of paths through which cortical effects to various brain stem neurones are conveyed and timing relations are determined.

CX – Cortex	MS – V Main Sensory Nucleus
VPM – Thalamic nucleus	ST – Supratrigeminal Nucleus
ventralis	R – Red Nucleus
posteromedialis	E – Facial Motoneurone
V Mes – V Mes. Tract Nucleus	H – Hypoglossal Motoneurone
JO – Jaw-opener Motoneurone	MOI – Inhibitory neurone in medial Reticular
JC – Jaw-closer Motoneurone	Formation

From these results, it appears that jaw muscles are represented in the face motor cortex in a qualitatively similar fashion to the hand muscle representation, and that flexor facilitation predominates over extensor facilitation. But jaw muscle representation is quantitatively different from that for arm muscles, that is, the innervation is not so strong as that for hand and tongue muscles.

CORTICOFUGAL CONNECTIONS

Figure 2 and Table 1 schematically summarize results of several microelectrode studies of synaptic effects from frontal cortex on brain stem neurones.

Facilitation or excitatory postsynaptic potentials (EPSPs) have been seen in digastric, masseteric, facial, and hypoglossal motoneurones (Porter, 1967; Chase et al., 1973; Clark and Luschei, 1974) and inhibition or inhibitory postsynaptic potentials (IPSPs) in masseter and facial motoneurones (Nakamura, Goldberg, and Clemente, 1967; Limansky et al., 1971). Chase and McGinty (1970a,b) showed in the chronic, unanaesthetized cat that digastric muscle

TABLE 1 A list of studies of cortical influences on brain stem neurones with the use of microelectrodes (see details in text). Columns indicate neuronal type, species used, shortest latency from the cortex (in msec), kind of potentials recorded, and name and year of author(s)

Neuronal type	Species	Latency (msec)	Potentials	Author(s)	Year
Digastric	Cat	10	(reflex)	Chase and McGinty	1970a
	Cat	5.4–7.6	(EPSP)	Limansky et al.	1971
	Squirrel monkey	6	(reflex)	Chase et al.	1973
	Rhesus monkey	8	(EMG)	Clark and Luschei	1974
Masseter	Cat	6	(IPSP)	Nakamura et al.	1967
	Squirrel monkey	4	(reflex)	Chase et al.	1973
	Rhesus monkey	8	(EMG)	Clark and Luschei	1974
Facial	Cat	5–6	(EPSP)	Wessolossky et al.	1968
	Cat	6.4	(EPSP)	Limansky et al.	1972
		7.5–10.0	(IPSP)		
	Cat	8.6	(EMG)	Woody	1974
Hypoglossal	Cat	8.5	(EPSP)	Porter	1967
V Primary afferent	Cat	20	(PD)	Dubner and Sessle	1971
V Main sensory nucleus	Cat	20	(PD)	Sessle and Dubner	1971
V Mes. tract nucleus	Cat	20	(PD)	Sauerland and Mizuno	1969

facilitation occurs in association with masseteric depression after orbital gyrus stimulation. The time course of digastric facilitation was from 10 to 20 msec or more, corresponding in time to an inhibitory effect in masseter motoneurones. Limansky et al. (1971) attempted intracellular recordings of digastric motoneurones during stimulation of somatosensory cortex, but the exact location of the stimulated site and stimulus parameters were not described. They recorded an EPSP with a latency of 5–6 msec in the anaesthetized cat. Wessolossky, Mizuno, and Clemente (1968) recorded intracellularly from facial motoneurones after shocks to orbital gyrus. They obtained EPSPs with a time course similar to the digastric facilitation. Limansky's group also tried intracellular recording from the facial motor nucleus (Limansky et al., 1972) and recorded EPSPs as well as IPSPs. The stimulated site was only described as the sensory-motor cortex. Porter (1967) recorded EPSPs (latency 8 msec) from hypoglossal motoneurones in the anaesthetized cat. Stimulated sites were the rostral portion of the lateral bank of the coronal gyrus.

Thus in motoneurones such as digastric, facial and hypoglossal, stimulation of the orbital gyrus or its adjacent areas evokes an excitatory effect. Simultaneously IPSPs are evoked in masseter motoneurones. The area capable of inducing cranial muscle contractions extends far laterally to the rostral part of the orbital gyrus. Therefore, the exact localization of the face motor area or cortical masticatory area must be determined. In view of the latency values of both EPSPs and IPSPs, the motoneurones seem to be activated indirectly from corticofugal fibres. Cortical inhibitory effects upon masseter motoneurones are abolished by making a transverse lesion at the lower pontine level, slightly caudal to the trigeminal motor nucleus (Sauerland et al., 1967). Nakamura, Takatori, and Kikuchi (1974) believe that an inhibitory interneurone for masseteric inhibition is located in the inhibitory zone of Magoun and Rhines (1946), to which terminal degeneration can be traced from the orbital gyrus (Mizuno, Sauerland, and Clemente, 1968). Also, the tegmentum, and particularly the supratrigeminal area, shows abundant terminal degenerations after removal of the monkey cortical masticatory area (Kuypers, 1958, 1960; Kidokoro et al., 1968a,b).

Presynaptic inhibition may contribute to cortically evoked effects. Presynaptic inhibitory (PD) effects start relatively slowly (see Table 1), and at present the functional significance of the cortically evoked presynaptic inhibitory phenomena is uncertain (cf. Sauerland and Mizuno, 1969; Dubner and Sessle, 1971; Sessle and Dubner, 1971).

In mastication, alpha-gamma linkage is expected to be important, yet it is noteworthy that we have had no basic anatomical and physiological studies clearly indicating the presence or characteristics of a gamma motor system in mastication until recently (see paper by Greenwood and Sessle, this volume).

Previous indications of its presence, though indirect, come from studies of jaw muscle spindle unit activity in voluntary or semi-automatic movements of the jaw (Matsunami and Kubota, 1972; Taylor and Cody, 1974). Matsunami and Kubota (1972) showed an increased unit activity during the shortening phase of the jaw-closing muscles. This was interpreted as resulting from increased fusimotor activity.

CORTICAL NEURONAL MECHANISMS

Knowledge of neuronal activities in the precentral cortex would provide important information of the cortico-brain stem loop in the control of mastication and swallowing. Three different groups, independent of each other, have recorded single unit activities in the monkey precentral cortex with reference to jaw movement. From the complicated array of jaw movements, jaw closing and jaw opening were primarily chosen and correlations made with the single unit activity. Luschei, Garthwaite, and Armstrong (1971) recorded unit activity from the face motor cortex when the monkey closed the jaw on presentation of a light signal. Kubota and Niki (1971) monitored neurones from the face motor area while the monkey was eating a small piece of apple, and recently Lund and Lamarre (1974) recorded units from the more lateral part of the precentral cortex while the monkey was chewing or making rhythmical 'tasting' movements.

The area searched by Luschei's group is roughly included within the face motor area, and corresponds to areas 6 and 4, mostly area 6 (Fig. 3). Also indicated in Figure 3 is the area searched by Kubota and Niki (1971). This region occupies the medial part of the cortical area studied by Luschei et al. and corresponds mostly to area 4 and partly to area 6. They found neuronal activity correlated to jaw activity at locations 4-6 mm laterally from the sites where they found units related to shoulder, hand, or arm movements. The area searched by Lund and Lamarre is located further laterally and includes areas 6a, 6b, 3a, and 3b.

Units related to jaw closing were found by Luschei et al. and Kubota and Niki. The highest activity was seen in the early phase of closing. More than half of the units were active just before the onset of the jaw-closing movement, as judged from the masseteric EMG or mechanical displacement of the jaw. Kubota and Niki suggested that these units may be related to initiation of jaw-closing movements. But the activity prior to the onset of jaw closing was not so striking as that seen in pyramidal tract neurones (PTN) of the hand or arm area. In the hand PTNs, such a weak coupling was not recognized and preceding activity was always present (Evarts et al., 1971). Luschei et al. (1971) suggested two possibilities: a motor interpretation hypothesis, or a

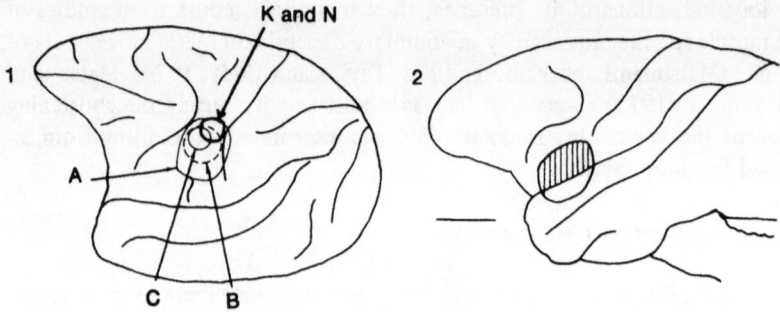

FIGURE 3 Lateral views of the monkey brain. Areas searched in single unit studies related to jaw movement.
1. Reproduced from Luschei et al. *J. Neurophysiol.* 34: 552–61 (1971). Courtesy of the author and publisher. Three circles (A, B, and C) indicated areas with units slightly (A), moderately (B), and heavily (C) concentrated. Thick circle with K & N indicates the area searched by Kubota and Niki (1971).
2. An area (oblique lines) searched by Lund and Lamarre (1974). Reproduced from Lund and Lamarre, *Exp. Brain Res.* 19: 282–99 (1974). Courtesy of the author and publisher.

somato-sensory modulation hypothesis, and either possibility was not excluded. Clark and Luschei's (1974) data of microstimulation strongly supports the view that there is a pathway from the motor cortex to the trigeminal motor nucleus, responsible for contraction of masseter and digastric muscles. It seems reasonable now to assume that unit activity in association with jaw closing may be coupled to the excitation of jaw-closing motoneurones. Activity preceding the movement may possibly provide excitatory and inhibitory influences to other parts, e.g. presynaptic inhibitory effects on the trigeminal mesencephalic tract nucleus, other brain stem sensory nuclei, and thalamic relay nuclei (Sauerland and Mizuno, 1969; Dubner and Sessle, 1971; Sessle and Dubner, 1971). The concept of 'corollary discharge,' proposed by Teuber to be a function of the prefrontal cortex and by Sperry or von Holst for optokinetic nystagmus (cf. Evarts et al., 1971), might also explain this neuronal activity.

As for units related to jaw opening, activity before the onset of the opening was seen in a small number of units by Kubota and Niki (the experimental arrangement used by Luschei's group did not allow detection of such discharges). In some jaw-opening units the preceding activity was only seen in initial trials of jaw opening during a series of jaw movements. This pattern may be comparable to the weakly phasic jaw-opening units described by Lund and Lamarre and resembles their tongue unit activity (cf. Fig. 7A of Lund and Lamarre, 1974). The preceding activity seen only in early series of trials in a rhythmic movement was not reported by others and therefore its correlation to jaw opening has yet to be confirmed.

Lund and Lamarre's data show that units in area 6b are complexly involved in mastication and swallowing and it is noteworthy that many units were activated from the periphery. Areas searched by them included the sensory cortex (e.g. areas 3a, 3b, and 1), so it might be expected that discharges recorded would be related to various sensory aspects of mastication and not necessarily show a correlation with the movement of the jaw. This sensory modulation may be involved in a more integrated manner with mastication and swallowing than with jaw closing and jaw opening. What kind of sensory inputs pass to this area must be determined and their roles in the initiation of movement clarified.

There has been little study of the sensory inputs to the cortex that eventually lead to masticatory and swallowing movements. It has been shown in acute experiments of cat and monkeys that cortical area 3a receives short-latency inputs from limb Group I afferents, probably from the muscle spindle. In the cat, area 3a for the face is wide (Hassler and Muhs-Clement, 1964), and it would be of interest to determine the kinds of inputs to this area.

REFERENCES

Asanuma, H., and Sakata, H. 1967. Functional organization of a cortical efferent system examined with focal depth stimulation in cats. *J. Neurophysiol.* 30: 35–54

Chase, M.H., and McGinty, D.J. 1970a. Modulation of spontaneous and reflex activity of the jaw musculature by orbital cortical stimulation in the freely-moving cat. *Brain Res.* 19: 117–26

— 1970b. Somatomotor inhibition and excitation by forebrain stimulation during sleep and wakefulness: orbital cortex. *Brain Res.* 19: 127–36

Chase, M.H., Sterman, M.B., Kubota, K., and Clemente, C.D. 1973. Modulation of masseteric and digastric neural activity by stimulation of the dorsolateral cerebral cortex in the squirrel monkey. *Exp. Neurol.* 41: 277–89

Clark, R.W., and Luschei, E.S. 1974. Short latency jaw movement produced by low intensity intracortical microstimulation of the precentral face area in monkeys. *Brain Res.* 70: 144–7

Dubner, R., and Sessle, B.J. 1971. Presynaptic excitability changes of primary afferent and corticofugal fibers projecting to trigeminal brain stem nuclei. *Exp. Neurol.* 30: 223–38

Evarts, E.V., Bizzi, E., Burke, R.E., Delong, M., and Thach, Jr., W.T. 1971. Central control of movement. *Neurosc. Res. Prog. Bull.* 9: 1–170

Ferrier, D. 1876. *The Functions of the Brain.* London: Smith, Elder & Co.

Green, H.D., and Walker, A.E. 1938. The effects of ablation of the cortical motor face area in monkeys. *J. Neurophysiol.* 1: 262–80

Hassler, R., and Muhs-Clement, K. 1964. Architektonischer Aufbau des senso-motorischen und parietalen Cortex der Katze. *J. Hirnforsch.* 6: 377–420

Hast, M.H., Fischer, J.M., Wetzel, A.B., and Thompson, V.E. 1974. Cortical motor representation of the laryngeal muscles in macaca mulatta. *Brain Res.* 73: 229–40

Hines, M. 1940. Movements elicited from precentral gyrus of adult chimpan-zees by stimulation with sine wave currents. *J. Neurophysiol.* 3: 442–66

Kaada, B.R. 1951. Somato-motor, autonomic and electrocorticographic responses to electrical stimulation of rhinencephalic and other structures in primates, cat and dog. *Acta physiol. scand.* 24. suppl. 83: 1–285

Kawamura, Y. 1964. Recent concepts of the physiology of mastication. In P.H. Staple (ed.), *Advances in Oral Biology.* Vol. 1. New York: Academic Press

Kidokoro, Y., Kubota, K., Shuto, S., and Sumino, R. 1968a. Reflex organiza-tion of cat masticatory muscles. *J. Neurophysiol.* 31: 695–708

– 1968b. Possible interneurons responsible for reflex inhibition of moto-neurons of jaw-closing muscles from the inferior dental nerve. *J. Neuro-physiol.* 31: 709–16

Kubota, K., and Niki, H. 1971. Precentral cortical unit activity and jaw move-ment in chronic monkeys. In R. Dubner and Y. Kawamura (eds.), *Oral-Facial Sensory and Motor Mechanisms.* New York: Appleton-Century-Crofts

Kuypers, H.G.J.M. 1958. Some projections from the pericentral cortex to the pons and lower brain stem in monkey and chimpanzee. *J. comp. Neurol.* 110: 221–56

– 1960. Central cortical projections to motor and somatosensory cell groups. *Brain* 83: 161–85

Lauer, E.W. 1952. Ipsilateral facial representation in motor cortex of macaque. *J. Neurophysiol.* 15: 1–4

Leyton, A.S.F., and Sherrington, C.S. 1917. Observations on the excitable cortex of the chimpanzee, orang-utan and gorilla. *Quart. J. exp. Physiol.* 11: 135–222

Limansky, Y.P., Pilyavsky, A.I., and Gura, E.V. 1971. Corticofugal influences on the trigeminal motoneurons. *Neirofiziologiia* 3: 512–19

– 1972. Postsynaptic potentials of facial motoneurons evoked by afferent and corticofugal volleys. *Neirofiziologiia* 4: 391–400

Lund, J.P., and Lamarre, Y. 1974. Activity of neurons in the lower precentral cortex during voluntary and rhythmical jaw movements in the monkey. *Exp. Brain Res.* 19: 282–99

Luschei, E.S., Garthwaite, C.R., and Armstrong, M.E. 1971. Relationship of firing patterns of units in face area of monkey precentral cortex to condi-tioned jaw movements. *J. Neurophysiol.* 34: 552–61

Magoun, H.W., and Rhines, R. 1946. An inhibitory mechanism in the bulbar reticular formation. *J. Neurophysiol.* 9: 165–71

Matsunami, K., and Kubota, K. 1972. Muscle afferents of trigeminal mesencephalic tract nucleus and mastication in chronic monkeys. *Jap. J. Physiol.* 22: 545–55

Mizuno, N., Sauerland, E.K., and Clemente, C.D. 1968. Projections from the orbital gyrus in the cat. I. To brain structures. *J. comp. Neurol.* 133: 463–75

Nakamura, Y., Goldberg, L.J., and Clemente, C.D. 1967. Nature of suppression of the masseteric monosynaptic reflex induced by stimulation of the orbital gyrus of the cat. *Brain Res.* 6: 184–98

Nakamura, Y., Takatori, S., and Kikuchi, J. 1974. Influences of medullary reticular formation upon the trigeminal motor neurons. Proc. 51st meeting Jap. Physiol. Soc. A–118. p.27

O'Brien, J.H., Pimpaneau, A., and Albe-Fessard, D. 1971. Evoked cortical responses to vagal, laryngeal and facial afferents in monkeys under chloralose anaesthesia. *Electroenceph. clin. Neurophysiol.* 31: 7–20

Porter, R. 1967. Cortical actions on hypoglossal motoneurones in cats: a proposed role for common internuncial cell. *J. Physiol. (Lond.)* 193: 295–308

Sauerland, E.K., Knauss, T., Nakamura, Y., and Clemente, C.D. 1967. Inhibition of monosynaptic and polysynaptic reflexes and muscle tone by electrical stimulation of the cerebral cortex. *Exp. Neurol.* 17: 159–71

Sauerland, E.K., and Mizuno, N. 1969. Cortically induced presynaptic inhibition of trigeminal proprioceptive afferents. *Brain Res.* 13: 556–68

Sauerland, E.K., Nakamura, Y., and Clemente, C.D. 1967. The role of the lower brain stem in cortically induced inhibition of somatic reflexes in the cat. *Brain Res.* 6: 164–80

Sessle, B.J., and Dubner, R. 1971. Presynaptic excitability changes of trigeminothalamic and corticothalamic afferents. *Exp. Neurol.* 30: 239–50

Sherrington, C. 1947. *The Integrative Action of the Nervous System.* New Haven: Yale Univ. Press

Stoney, Jr., S.D., Thompson, W.D., and Asanuma, H. 1968. Excitation of pyramidal tract cells by intracortical microstimulation: effective extent of stimulating current. *J. Neurophysiol.* 31: 659–69

Sumi, T. 1969. Some properties of cortically-evoked swallowing and chewing in rabbits. *Brain Res.* 15: 107–20

Taylor, A., and Cody, F.W.J. 1974. Jaw muscle spindle activity in the cat during normal movements of eating and drinking. *Brain Res.* 71: 523–30

Tsukamoto, S. 1963. Studies on brain mechanisms of jaw movements: I. Analysis of jaw movements from the cortical jaw motor area and amygdala in the rabbit. *J. Physiol. Soc. Jap.* 25: 12–24 (In Japanese)

Vogt, O., and Vogt, C. 1919. Ergebnisse unserer Hirnforchung. *J. Psychol. Neurol.* (Lpz.) 25: 277–462

Von Bonin, G. 1949. Architecture of the precentral motor cortex and some
    adjacent areas. In P.C. Bucy (ed.), *The Precentral Motor Cortex.* Urbana,
    Ill.: Univ. Illinois Press
Walker, A.E., and Green H.D. 1938. Electrical excitability of the motor face
    area: a comparative study in primates. *J. Neurophysiol.* 1: 152-65
Wessolossky, J., Mizuno, N., and Clemente, C.D. 1968. Effect of orbital corti-
    cal stimulation upon the facial motoneurons of the cat. *Fed. Proc.* 27: 451
Woody, C.D. 1974. Aspects of the electrophysiology of cortical processes
    related to the development and performance of learned motor responses.
    Physiologist 17: 49-70
Woolsey, C.N., Settlage, P.H., Meyer, D.R., Sencer, W., Pinto Hamuy, T.,
    and Travis, A.M. 1952. Patterns of localization in precentral and 'supple-
    mentary' motor areas and their relation to the concept of a premotor area.
    Res. Publ. Ass. nerv. ment. Dis. 30: 238-64

DISCUSSION

SESSLE   In acute experiments in cats, Dr Lund and I recently described a
Group I jaw muscle afferent projection to cortex (J.P. Lund and B.J. Sessle,
Exp. Neurol. 45 [1974]: 314-31). But your excellent review of the present
state of the art, particularly with respect to cortical cell activity and mastication and swallowing, does emphasize the value of the chronic experimental
approach. Nevertheless, I think you would agree that some caution is required
in interpreting the function of these cortical cells. Much of their 'functional
role' is based upon the temporal nature of their discharge in relation to, for
example, an electromyographic response. However, we do not really know
whether these cells are necessarily 'hooked up' to the motoneurones concerned, either directly or indirectly. We do know from anatomical studies
that some of these cells project down to the brain stem, and I am reminded in
the work by Evarts and others that you mention that, with movements of the
limb, there are cells in the basal ganglia, cerebellum, cortex, and thalamic
nuclei all of which may fire in advance of the movement. One could implicate
these as the cause of the movement, but this is not necessarily the case.
LUND   Some of the cells which we record do have a very nice relationship between the firing pattern and the first part of the movement, particularly jaw
opening. It is true that they are not easy to find. I would also like to mention
the experiments we have been carrying out using cortical stimulation in the
awake monkey. When we stimulated the bottom of area 4, we obtained tongue and facial movements. Single shocks gave a twitch of the contralateral
face, and a slight movement of the tongue. As we moved across we started to

see repetitive jaw movements using a stimulus of 60 Hz and about 5-9 μA intensity. However, these were not very natural, and mainly ipsilateral. As we came towards the subcentral dimple, we obtained very natural movements bilaterally, and with good coordination between the facial muscles and tongue muscles.

KUBOTA Where do you think this area is?

LUND Probably near area 6b.

SESSLE Why do you think you have to give such large repetitive stimuli to elicit these sorts of effects? We now know that if one gets inside some of these cells or near them, movements can occur with low stimulus strengths.

LUND The stimulation currents we used were not very high, under 10 μA.

SESSLE But you are using very high frequencies. What does this mean in terms of natural mechanisms? Presumably internuncial chains of neurones are implicated.

LUND Yes, it is not the cortical cell that you have to stimulate at that high a frequency since you can obtain the same effect by stimulating the cortical tract. I think that to produce the repetitive masticatory pattern, you have to have spatial and temporal summation in the brain stem.

SESSLE As you go down from cortex to the brain stem in the same animal, is there a decrease in the threshold or stimulus parameters required to elicit the movements? You might expect that as the stimulus is applied closer and closer to this area, less intense stimulation may be necessary.

KAWAMURA We find that we need less stimulation in the brain stem than in the amygdala to produce the same effect.

DUBNER Here we are undoubtedly dealing with a number of synapses before we get to the jaw motoneurones. This contrasts with the pathways to some muscles in the primate where descending neurones make monosynaptic connections with the motoneurones. It fits in quite well with the idea that one needs to have spatial and temporal summation to produce a response, and that it is difficult to obtain responses from the areas stimulated by Kubota and Luschei.

HANNAM How feasible is it to use multiple stimulation techniques, for example using microstimulation of several different sites at the same time? For example, one could produce combinations of inputs from different areas and observe the effects of their interactions.

LUND I believe Sumi (1969) did some experiments in which he stimulated the masticatory areas in both hemispheres to show summation effects.

GOBEL Are there species differences with regard to the projections from the cortex to cranial motor nuclei?

KUBOTA There is a difference between chimpanzee and rhesus monkey in degeneration studies involving projections to trigeminal, facial, and hypoglossal nuclei (Kuypers, 1958).

GOBEL These corticofugal projections to the brain stem and spinal cord are very weak, despite the fact that the Fink-Heimer pictures look good. There are very few endings/unit length of axon. We find this sort of thing in the trigeminal sensory nuclei, and it could explain why you have some trouble driving motoneurones. This contrasts with corticothalamic projections, where there is a much greater density of endings.

KUBOTA Dr Lund, you have seen contralateral movements on stimulation. Have you also seen ipsilateral movements as well? By dividing the symphysis of the jaw, Leyton and Sherrington (1917) noted that cortical representation is mainly unilateral.

LUND The movements which we saw were either ipsilateral face, jaw, or tongue movements, or bilateral rhythmical movements.

SUMI I have stimulated the motor area, recorded from hypoglossal motoneurones, and measured the latency of the response (T. Sumi, *Pflügers Arch.* 314 [1970]: 329-46). Here is another group of neurones which do not produce a response in the first 5 msec or so, although when they do respond they do so in a rhythmical fashion. I would like to stress how important it is to take note of the effect of anaesthesia in this sort of study.

GREENWOOD Is there any anatomical or physiological evidence that the excitation of these cortical neurones has an inhibitory influence on neuronal processes in the trigeminal nuclei?

KUBOTA It is clear that there is a presynaptic inhibitory mechanism from the cortex to the brain stem neurones (e.g. Sauerland and Mizuno, 1969; Sessle and Dubner, 1971).

DUBNER In many of the experiments we are talking about, the animal has been trained to perform repetitive, stereotyped movements, and attempts are made to relate movement, behaviour, and neuronal discharge. Even here, it is often extremely difficult to pin-point what the relationship is. When we consider studies carried out on animals involved in chewing, we are looking at many muscles in function, and at movements that are not stereotyped. This presents great problems. I think one of the things we must do is try to define the movement that takes place in the jaw area, and perhaps train animals to perform more stereotyped movements.

STOREY I wonder whether cortical stimulation may in some cases disrupt other cortical activity that is occurring, and so mask other neural events. I would also be interested to hear any comments regarding the possibility of a cortical mechanism for controlling the transition between chewing and swallowing rather than a brain stem mechanism. If there is some organization going on in the cortex, then the swallow threshold may well be determined in the cortex as a result of learning.

SESSLE The fact that both chewing and swallowing can be produced by brain stem stimulation would suggest that the cortex does not exercise a profound influence. We are not sure, of course, whether the same area in the brain stem is responsible for the coordination of chewing and swallowing.

KUBOTA High-voltage, high-frequency stimulation is very disruptive. As a result many indirect effects are possible. With regard to the second point made by Dr Storey, we tried to induce swallowing by microstimulation of the cortex and did not succeed, so the argument for brain stem coordination would be supported.

STOREY I wonder whether the level of anaesthetic during cortical stimulation would have any effect on the chewing-swallowing sequence, whether swallowing might drop out, for example, and chewing remain.

SUMI Yes, chewing drops out first (Sumi, 1969).

MATTHEWS Dr Kubota, what were your criteria for the identification of muscle spindles?

KUBOTA We gave a single shock to the semilunar ganglion in the jaw-opened state to elicit a silent phase in the unit activity, while the jaw-closing muscles were contracting. We did not measure the conduction velocity of the unit.

MATTHEWS So you think you are stimulating motor axons as they pass below the semilunar ganglion?

KUBOTA Yes. This silent phase is very short (10–20 msec), compared with that in the limb muscles. Therefore, we have to test at the jaw-opened state by passive stretching.

SESSLE Could not some of these units be interneurones near or even in the mesencephalic nucleus, which have a muscle spindle and, say, a trigeminal cutaneous input; thus when you stimulate the trigeminal ganglion you might conceivably be producing an orthodromically induced inhibition?

KUBOTA That possibility is not completely excluded, although the neurones which we have found have been within the nucleus. To exclude this possibility, it is necessary first to measure the conduction velocity and second to determine the relation between stimulus intensity and the induced silent phase. The second point is difficult to examine in the chronic unanaesthetized state because single unit activity is lost by movement.

SESSLE Anatomical studies have indicated that there may be neurones in the nucleus which are not primary afferent cell bodies (e.g. G.E. Foster, *J. Anat. (Lond.)* 114 [1973] : 293; J.E. Hubbard, and V. Di Carlo, *J. comp. Neurol.* 147 [1973] : 553–66).

Chairman's Summary

B.J. SESSLE

In this section, we have identified the reflex and higher centre control mechanisms occurring on oral-facial motoneurones involved in mastication and swallowing. To what extent these controls operate during mastication and swallowing is debatable, but the session has provided a good basis for those remaining sessions and workshops that deal with the ways in which mastication and swallowing are laid down. The reflex inputs to the motoneurones are numerous and varied, and the type and pattern of these inputs and their influences show many fundamental differences from those studied so extensively (e.g. Eccles, 1964; Matthews, 1972) in spinal motoneurones. Because of the complex nature of mastication and swallowing compared with spinal motility patterns, it is probably not too surprising that differences exist. I think it worthwhile to summarize some of these:

(a) The cell bodies of jaw muscle spindle afferents are located *within* the central nervous system, in the trigeminal mesencephalic nucleus. Synaptic profiles are seen here (e.g. Alley, 1973), but their origins and function (modulating, neurotrophic, etc.) are uncertain.

(b) There is an apparent lack of low-threshold muscle afferents in many cranial motor nerves.

(c) Muscle spindles and their central influences are absent in many muscles. Thus reciprocal innervation, so fundamental a concept at the spinal level and an important mechanism contributing to posture and locomotion, is extremely limited at the brain stem level. Other mechanisms must exist to account for the variety of motility patterns required for mastication, swallowing, and associated movements, and these are considered in the workshop reports.

(d) The Golgi tendon organ and its central influences are an important depressive influence of spinal motoneurone activity. Is the lack of evidence of these receptors in the oral-facial region real, or a reflection of a lack of careful study? Are they not needed because other inhibitory mechanisms exist (periodontal, mucosal, etc.) which make their presence superfluous? Perhaps their role at spinal levels is related to reciprocal innervation and locomotion, and this mechanism is not required as a substrate for mastication and swallowing. Some recent unpublished data reported by Dr Lund in his presentation suggests in fact that Golgi tendon organs may occur in jaw muscles, so clarification of their existence and function may be imminent.

(e) Only a *limited* gamma motoneurone system occurs in the cranial nerves. Recently, firm evidence for the system has been provided, at least for the jaw-closing muscles (see paper by Greenwood and Sessle, this volume). The scarcity of muscle spindles and thus a gamma system associated with other muscles may occur because the muscles of the tongue, face, pharynx, larynx, etc. do not require such an elaborate feedback control in the types of movements that they are concerned with in subprimates. But what is role of the gamma system in masticatory function? What sorts of peripheral and central influences play onto this system? How do the alpha-gamma systems interact in voluntary and involuntary jaw movements and in mastication? Is there alpha-gamma coactivation, or gamma leading? Evidence so far suggests the former, but recordings from both types of motoneurones in the chronic awake animal would be an approach that should help answer this and other related questions.

It is obvious from our discussions that there has been little use made of the effects of natural stimuli in reflex control mechanisms, particularly utilizing stimuli of the type that might occur in normal masticatory and deglutitory functions. Moreover, most of the studies of central, and especially peripheral, controls have been carried out in subprimates. Can the results of these be extrapolated and the findings applied to neural mechanisms operative in the human? Experiments on monkeys probably offer the closest approach we can make, although some of the reflex effects noted in subprimates have been identified in humans, e.g. tooth-tap inhibition of the jaw-closing muscles can be obtained experimentally in humans as well as in the cat. But whether such reflex effects provide the basis for chewing must, on the basis of recent evidence, now be considered unlikely, as pointed out by Dr Goldberg and in the first workshop report. The full significance of the variety of inhibitory and facilitatory influences from the periphery awaits further study.

Many of the inhibitory and facilitatory influences on motoneurone activity can also be elicited from suprasegmental sites such as cerebral cortex. Do long-loop 'reflexes' involving brain stem and cortex contribute to the motoneuronal processes underlying mastication and swallowing? Evidence is accumulating, particularly from chronic experiments on the frontal cortex, of its contribution to sensorimotor integration and voluntary control of masticatory and deglutitory movements. Such approaches auger well for future advances in our knowledge of higher control mechanisms.

But what of other suprasegmental controls? Dr Kubota has mentioned that many other central sites, at a gross level, can influence oral-facial motility. How are such effects achieved? What is the contribution of these centres and their controls in the development and learning of oral-facial motility patterns? What is the importance of their interaction with the reflex inputs in the acquisition of these patterns? Motoneurone studies in the developing as well as the mature animal are crucial for such answers. In fact, I think it is fair to conclude that correlation of the biological and clinical aspects of mastication and swallowing cannot be satisfactorily achieved until the central neuronal mechanisms of reflex and suprasegmental controls are further elucidated.

REFERENCES

Alley, K.E. 1973. Quantitative analysis of the synaptogenic period in the trigeminal mesencephalic nucleus. *Anat. Rec.* 177: 49–60
Eccles, J.C. 1964. *The Physiology of Synapses.* Berlin: Springer
Matthews, P.B.C. 1972. *Mammalian Muscle Receptors and Their Central Actions.* London: Arnold

SECTION THREE

Mastication and swallowing:
Pain and related sensory influences

Chairman's Introduction

R. DUBNER

Pain is a complex sensory experience. It involves our sensory capacities to discriminate the quality, location, intensity, and duration of a noxious stimulus. Our perception of the stimulus and behavioural responses to it also involve those components of the central nervous system concerned with how we 'feel about the pain.' This includes factors such as previous experiences with pain, cultural background, personality, and present psychological state or set. In other words, pain reaction and response are greatly influenced by predisposing factors which provide a higher brain centre control over sensory sensitivity to tissue-threatening stimuli.

The problem of chronic pathological pain in humans reaches another level of complexity. In the extreme, there are patients who suffer persistent or intermittent pain with no apparent stimulation. In most cases of pathological pain, however, we have some knowledge of the aetiologic and stimulus factors which evoke the pain response. For instance, in classical cases of trigeminal neuralgia, a great deal is known about the quality, location, and other stimulus parameters which can produce paroxysmal episodes of pain. The peripheral and central nervous system pathology responsible for this effect unfortunately is poorly understood. The myofascial, or temporomandibular joint, pain-dysfunction syndrome is another chronic pain problem where we know something about the site of origin of the pain but little about mechanisms. In this syndrome, pain arises from muscle sites, in general, and very often the jaw-closing masticatory muscles are involved. What peripheral or central nervous system changes produce pathological muscle activity with resultant muscle pain? Do sensory impulses from teeth, periodontal membrane, temporomandibular joint, and muscle itself play a role in producing this pathological state? Are predisposing psychological factors significant contributors to a central excitatory state which augments aberrant muscle activity?

These are questions that can be answered if we examine in isolation some of the reflex activity concerned with mandibular posture and jaw movements.

Jaw-opening muscles are activated by a variety of innocuous or non-painful perioral and oral inputs including periodontal membrane, gingiva, and the temporomandibular joint. On the other hand, noxious input arising from teeth, periodontal membrane, and perioral structures produce a protective reflex with inhibition of the powerful jaw-closing muscles. Are such reflexes overridden by central excitation in oral-facial pain-dysfunction syndromes? It is also known, at spinal cord levels, that protective reflexes are evoked from muscle by activation of Group III and IV afferent fibres (Matthews, 1972). Such fibres are thought, in part, to be nociceptive, and these so-called flexor reflex afferents produce inhibition of antigravity muscles. Such protective reflexes involving the jaw musculature would produce inhibition of jaw-closing muscles. What peripheral and central neural factors are capable of overriding this important reflex?

It is clear that the control of jaw muscle activity involves multiple peripheral and central factors. Central pathways that can provide these sensory interactions include the trigeminal brain stem nuclear complex, other cranial sensory nuclei, the reticular nuclei, and descending pathways that converge on these centres.

During this section we shall examine the anatomical organization and functional relationships of brain stem nuclei involved in oral-facial reflex activity. Our understanding of pathological pain syndromes in the oral-facial area is dependent on knowledge of the basic neuronal circuitry responsible for the modulation of trigeminal motoneurone activity. This section will help us establish the present state of knowledge and set forth future research goals.

REFERENCE

Matthews, P.B.C. 1972. *Mammalian Muscle Receptors and their Central Actions.* Baltimore: Williams and Wilkins

Mandibular dysfunction or jaw-related headaches: a review and definition

R.H. ROYDHOUSE

The literature associated with facial and head pain reflects the confusion of Alice in Wonderland, who thought that 'I mean what I say' was the same as 'I say what I mean,' and in a similar sense, paraphrasing the Mad Hatter's remarks, the phrases 'I see what I treat' and 'I treat what I see' have guided much of the literature.

Wright (1920) hoped his paper on jaw position and deafness as a result would lead to clarity, but later Roberts (1936) said 'One of my greatest difficulties has been getting the co-operation of dentists.' Finneson (1969), in reference to temporomandibular joint (TMJ) pain observed that dentists tended to be 'over-aggressive in the treatment of the problem,' and Greene (1973) who asked dentists, oral surgeons, and medical practitioners about the myofascial* pain dysfunction syndrome noted the 'chaotic situation that prevails among current practitioners.'

The present situation has recently been summarized by De Boever (1973). He described twelve different names that have been applied to the disorder and stated that the 'over-abundance of terms is confusing.' His review of present ideas and treatment methods provides an overall view of traditional approaches. Hilton in 1863 was clear and direct. He said that opium introduced into the auditory canals relieves toothache and stiff jaws.

SURVEYS

In answer to the editorial question (Macdonald, 1972) 'Are the data worth owning?,' the reply was 'usually an embarrassing and costly "no" ... the problem lies in the lack of knowledge about the trustworthiness of the data.' Such seems to be the case with most surveys because the criteria of selection and definitions of the symptoms are not given.

*Sometimes referred to as 'myofacial.'

TABLE 1   Occurrence of reports of pain, symptoms, signs and aetiology from 11 surveys

	Pain				Other symptoms		Signs	Aetiology		
	Supra-orbital / Temporal	Cervical	Ear-TMJ	Mandibular	Stiff Jaw	Aural	TMJ click	Natural teeth	Partial loss	Dentures
Hankey, 1958	x	x	x	x	x			x	x	x
Gelb et al., 1967	x	x	x		x	x		x	x	x
Posselt, 1968*	x		x		x	x	x			
Perry, 1968	x	x	x	x			x			
Roydhouse, N., 1968		x	x			x				
Greene, 1969	x	x			x	x	x			
Hupfauf and Weitkamp, 1969	x		x		x		x			
Thompson, 1971			x		x		x			
Duker et al., 1972			x				x		x	
Roydhouse, R.H., 1974	x	x	x	x	x	x	x	x	x	x
Thiel, 1970	x	x								
No. reporting	8	7	9	3	7	5	9	3	4	3

*Composite of others.

Table 1 catalogues signs and symptoms reported in 11 surveys of patients. Pain about the ear, the eyes, the temples and the neck are reported in most instances. A stiff jaw with temporomandibular grating or clicking, and aural symptoms other than pain (such as tinnitus, deafness, or other auditory effects) are also mentioned in the majority of reports.

Table 2 shows a calculation of the percentages of reported signs and symptoms, some of which are approximations gained from authors' bar graphs. In addition, mean values which are possibly fallacious have been calculated. Pain is the most frequent symptom. In Posselt's review (1968), the TMJ click is more significant. Gelb et al. (1967) and N. Roydhouse (1970) are associated with ear, nose, and throat institutions and consequently report mostly aural effects. Dizziness or vertigo is a concern of three reports only. Only Gelb et al. and R.H. Roydhouse report signs other than a TMJ click.

Table 3 represents a survey of patients seen in a private practice in Vancouver. This implies a certain socio-economic bias. Patients were referred mainly by physicians, and by dentists, who guessed or knew that the patients' complaints were related to jaw movements. Only 4 or 6 per cent were apparently free of pain. Aural effects such as sporadic deafness, plugged ears, and tinnitus, were present in 60 per cent, dizziness in 33 per cent, and excessive salivation and lacrimatory effects in over 20 per cent. Excessive salivation was con-

TABLE 2 Percentages reporting pain, other symptoms, signs, and possible aetiology

	Pain				Other symptoms						Signs			Aetiology factors					No. of patients
	Supra-orbital Temporal	Cervical	Ear-TMJ	Mandibular	Stiff Jaw	Aural	Dizziness	Salivation	Lacrimation	Optical	TMJ click	Internal Ptery.	Submand. Gland	Natural teeth	Partial loss	Dentures	Dental treat.	Accident	
Hankey, 1958	82	5	10	7	6	—	—	—	—	—	—	—	—	70	30	14	—	—	100
Gelb et al., 1967	20	10	35	—	4	42	—	—	—	—	18	81	—	20	70	10	—	—	742
Posselt, 1968*	6	—	14	—	17	10	—	—	—	—	30	—	—	—	—	—	—	—	467
Perry, 1968	68	41	98	47	—	—	—	—	—	—	73	—	—	—	—	—	—	—	40
Roydhouse, N., 1968	—	15	55	—	—	60	38	—	—	—	18	—	—	—	—	—	—	—	262
Greene, 1969	87	43	—	—	63	7	—	—	—	—	66	—	—	—	—	—	—	—	
Hupfauf and Weitkamp, 1969	36	—	62	—	62	—	—	—	—	—	62	—	—	—	—	—	—	—	235
Thompson, 1971	—	—	64	—	7	—	—	—	—	—	42	—	—	—	—	—	—	—	100
Duker et al., 1972	—	—	47	—	—	—	33	—	—	—	47	—	—	—	66	—	—	—	127
Roydhouse, R.H., 1974	65	70	58	12	22	58	33	32	20	32	38	76	56	27	10	20	15	33	60
Thiel, 1970 A	15	4	—	—	—	—	—	—	—	—	—	—	—	—	—	—	—	—	264
B	12	4	—	—	—	—	—	—	—	—	—	—	—	—	—	—	—	—	
Mean	52	31	49	22	25	35	34	32	20	32	44	79	56	40	44	15	15	33	

*Composite of many others.
Note. Group A are 'bruxists' and B are not.

TABLE 3   Mandibular dysfunction:
Survey of 60 patients (private practice)

Symptoms	Percentage noted
Location of pain	
Frontal	65
Occipital or cervical	70
Ear and/or TMJ	58
Mandibular	12
Patient-reported symptoms	
Stiffness of jaw	22
Aural deafness	58
Dizziness	33
Excessive salivation	32
Excessive lacrimation	20
Optical changes	32
Signs from clinical examination	
TMJ click	38
Internal pterygoid painful	76
Submandibular gland painful	56

sidered present when the patient noted difficulty with excessive saliva or reported that, during sleep at night, the pillow became saturated with saliva.

In this table, the signs are, in a sense, more important than the symptoms,
in that objectivity is more likely. Of particular interest is the high incidence
of painful submandibular glands, reported first in 1973 (Roydhouse). Of the
patients surveyed, two-thirds had either swollen glands or excessive lacrima-
tion, and only one-sixth had both. The internal pterygoid muscle is important
as a sign because it is remote, unrecognized by the patient, and can be differentiated from headaches. Pain in this muscle may be described under symptoms as a sore throat or swollen glands (Roydhouse, 1973).

As shown in Possibility B (Table 4), nearly half the patients had been associated with external events. The high percentage (70) with neck pains (Table
3) occurs because many of these patients had suffered rapid deceleration
effects (whiplash), and this affected their necks as well. In other surveys, it is
not possible to know what percentage of subjects had been in accidents as
'whiplash' has not been thought a possible causal agent. In the present survey,
psychological factors as causal agents were minor, and acute conditions, – viz.
accidents and dental treatment, – were major influences.

TABLE 4   Mandibular dysfunction: Suspected aetiology and
results of treatment – survey of 60 patients (private practice)
(all figures refer to percentages)

Possible aetiological factors described in two alternative ways
(both columns list relative frequencies occurring in the sample)

Possibility A		Possibility B	
Natural teeth	27	Car accident	33
Partial loss	10	Dental treatment	15
Dentures	20	Other	52
Car accident	33		100
Dental treatment	15		
Difficult personalities	18		

Results of treatment

Reported satisfactory one year later	73
Reported not satisfactory one year later	3
Not treated completely or not available	23

DEFINITIONS

A definition of a potential disorder can emerge despite the untrustworthiness
of the data. The definition is defined by symptoms, and is not based on aetiology because of the uncertainty of the links between original cause (if any
single one exists) and end-result. It is treatment-oriented; a disorder is established which can be treated by a variety of manipulations, either of the jaw
position, its movements or the structures which power or restrict the movements, that is muscles, teeth, and joints.

Thus mandibular dysfunction is that disorder of the jaw, associated muscles, joints, and teeth, and interrelated systems, which produces pain or dis-
comfort about the temples, the side of the head (particularly the ear), and
secondarily pain about the neck and lower jaw. Such pain is frequently associated with aural changes and it influences, or is influenced by, the autonomic
nervous system. Painful internal pterygoid muscles, swollen or painful submandibular glands and possible joint malfunction are accompanying signs.

DISCUSSION

Pain is the main symptom and the main motivation to seek treatment. Hilton
in 1863 offered the advice, particularly in regard to the trigeminal nerve, that
'if the hidden cause of pain be in any one particular spot, it is only by tracing

the nerves of and from that spot that we can hope to arrive logically at the real cause of the symptoms and so divest the cause of its obscurity.' An inspection of what could be called the 'wiring diagram' of the head and neck leaves the viewer not knowing which 'wire' or nerve or set of nerves is the source and which is the reflection, or the referred pain. Racial origin (Zobrowski, 1969), the patient's mental state (Yemm, 1969) before the onset (Friedman and Fraser, 1970) and after chronic pain (Timmermans and Sternbach, 1974), as well as the plurality of factors involved in head trauma (Nick and Sicard-Nick, 1969), make the seeking of causal links based upon the patient's appreciation of his disorder a hazardous logical task. In addition, the psychological or traditional bent of the investigator plays a role.

The pain of trigeminal neuralgia, it is asserted, is different to mandibular dysfunction pain, being supposedly always paroxysmal in nature. There is an artificial separation of 'trigeminal neuralgia' related to treatment and especially to the politics of treatment. If it can only be treated by resection of the sensory root of the fifth nerve, then it is apparently tic douloureux. Blair and Gordon (1973), Lindsay (1969), and I have found that persons diagnosed as cases of tic douloureux can be cured or have their symptoms abated by combined drug therapy and changes in mandibular posture. Kränzl and Kränzl (1973) suggested that irritation of the sympathetic nerves produces tic douloureux in the ophthalmic and maxillary divisions and of the parasympathetic in the mandibular division.

In fact, it is suggested that the aetiologies of tic douloureux, and the disorder defined above and usually described by De Boever's twelve names, are equally obscure. The definition proposed suggests pain related to mandibular function and does not specify a nerve, a set of nerves, or an aetiology. In the past, theories have been converted to facts by the circuitous logical fallacy noted by Sicuteri (1970).

Bruxism is similarly confused – is it a cause, a result, or an associated phenomenon (Thiel, 1970; Christensen, 1971; Molin, 1972; Lindquist and Ringquist, 1973)? The skulls of adult Indians, Maoris, and many other races, in fact most prehistoric peoples and present 'underdeveloped' races who lack refined foods and dentistry (Roydhouse and Simonsen, 1974), show signs of so-called bruxism. What appears to be bruxism may be normal activity of the mandibular articulation; it may be a normal function of man which has become restricted in civilized societies by dental treatment. The so-called psychologic ground in which the disorder is supposed to develop is likewise a possible cause-effect reversal. Patients presenting in a confused state after 6 to 12 months of pain could be suffering deprivation of REM sleep. Reding et al. (1968) noted that mandibular movements occur just before or during REM sleep.

TREATMENT CONSIDERATIONS

Each treatment is individual – both for operators and patients. Successful treatment depends upon the restoration of a dental occlusion on both sides which allows free or relatively unimpeded movements of the mandible when the teeth are together. Associated with this is the establishment of a jaw separation or muscle length or, in our jargon, a 'vertical dimension' which is symptomless. In some patients reputed to have this disorder, a reduction in overall muscle tension by drugs, placebos, and psychic manipulation will decrease and sometimes eliminate symptoms. It is not possible to say whether this style or that style is more successful, because the evidence is unavailable or untrustworthy. Hence the disparate reports that occur referring to the role of placebos, personality characteristics, feedback devices, and so on. Such research is confusing and creates the problem that Greene (1973) detected.

FUTURE NEEDS AND DIRECTIONS

Tinbergen (1974), in his Nobel prize acceptance speech, stated that 'the basic scientific method is still too often looked down on by those blinded by the glamour of apparatus, the prestige of tests, and by the temptation to turn to drugs.' In the address, he referred particularly to the field of somatic malfunction and psychosocial stress. It is possible to separate mandibular malfunction from other disorders as history and practical experience suggest. The greatest error to be made, and that has been made, is the assumption of aetiologies and thus of causal links. The very need for this conference indicates diversity of views, paucity of coordinated knowledge, and areas of unknown content and unknown importance. By 'watching and wondering,' as Berry (1969) puts it, a Natural History of Mandibular Dysfunction can be catalogued. The assumption should be that at the present time, the causal links that lead to the dysfunction are uncertain. Aetiology would be restricted to such visible unmistakeable categories as trauma, gross dental malformations, disease processes associated with the masticatory system, and unknown. Research and treatment should follow the usual pattern instead of being invested with mystery, suppositions, and notions (Nairn, 1974).

Finally in speculation, the individual significance and perhaps some aspects of aetiology may be discerned by regarding evolution; Darlington (1969) states that one of the four sets of behaviour building communities together and thus determining the genetic factor of man is speech, and this is 'the most important of all.' Are we not discussing the organ or system which distinguishes man from other animals? We all eat but only man speaks.

CONCLUSION

A disorder called mandibular dysfunction has been defined, based on clinical reports over the last 40 years and from the personal viewpoint of a clinician. By such a definition, the assumption of incorrect aetiologic factors should be avoided. By examination of patients and normal persons, the causal links leading to head pain and headaches associated with somatic malfunction of jaws and related structures may become clearer in time.

REFERENCES

Berry, D.C. 1969. Mandibular dysfunction pain and chronic minor illness. *Brit. dent. J.* 127: 170–5
Blair, G.A.S., and Gordon, D.S. 1973. Trigeminal neuralgia. *Brit. med. J.* 4: 38–40
Christensen, L.V. 1971. Facial pain and internal pressure of masseter muscle in experimental bruxism in man. *Archs oral Biol.* 16: 1021–31
Darlington, C.D. 1969. *The Evolution of Man and Society.* London: George Allen and Unwin
De Boever, J. 1973. Functional disturbances of the temporomandibular joints. *Oral Sciences Rev.* 2: 100–17
Duker, J., Philipp, U., and Fiebelkorn, W. 1972. Sensorische Storungen bei Kiefergelenkerkrankungen. *Deutsch. Zahnaerztl. Z.* 27: 811–5
Finneson, B.E. 1969. *Diagnosis and Management of Pain Syndrome.* Philadelphia: Saunders
Friedman, A.P., and Fraser, S.H. 1970. Preliminary observations of psychiatric evaluation of treated chronic headache patients. *Res. Clin. Stud. Headache* 3: 373–80
Gelb, H., Calderone, J.P., Gross, S.M., and Kantor, M.E. 1967. The role of the dentist and the otolaryngologist in evaluating temporomandibular joint syndromes. *J. prosth. Dent.* 18: 497–503
Greene, C.S. 1973. A survey of current professional concepts and opinions about myofascial pain-dysfunction (MPD) syndrome. *JADA* 86: 128–36
Hankey, G.T. 1958. Some observations on Costen's mandibular syndrome. *Proc. Roy. Soc. Med.* 51: 225–32
Hilton, J. 1863. *On the Influence of Mechanical and Physiological Rest in the Treatment of Accidents and Surgical Diseases and the Diagnostic Value of Pain.* London: Bill and Doldy
Hupfauf, L., and Weitkamp, J. 1969. Ergebnisse der Behandulung von funktionsbedingten Erkrankungen des Kausystems mit Aufbissplatten. *Deutsch. Zahnaerztl. Z.* 24: 347–52

Kränzl, B., and Kränzl, C. 1973. Neue Beiträge zue Therapie der trigeminus-neuralgie. *Osterr. Z. Stom.* 70: 54–64

Lindquist, B., and Ringquist, M. 1973. Bite force in children with bruxism. *Acta odont. scand.* 31: 255–9

Lindsay, B. 1969. Trigeminal neuralgia: a new approach. *Med. J. Austral.* 1: 8–13

Macdonald, J.R. 1972. Are the data worth owning? *Science* 176: 3

Molin, C. 1972. Vertical isometric muscle forces of the mandible: a comparative study of subjects with and without manifest mandibular pain dysfunction syndrome. *Acta odont. scand.* 30: 485–99

Nairn, R.I. 1974. Maxillomandibular relations and aspects of occlusion. *J. prosth. dent.* 31: 361–8

Nick, J., and Sicard-Nick, C. 1969. Chronic post-traumatic headache. *Res. Clin. Stud. Headache* 2: 115–68

Perry, H.T. 1968. The symptomology of temporomandibular joint disturbance. *J. prosth. dent.* 19: 288–98

Posselt, U. 1968. *Physiology of Occlusion and Rehabilitation.* Oxford: Blackwell

Reding, G.R., Zepelin, H., Robinson, J.E., Zimmerman, S.O., and Smith, V.H. 1968. Nocturnal teeth-grinding: all-night psychophysiologic studies. *J. dent. Res.* 47: 786–97

Roberts, S. 1936. Cited in Costen, J.B. 1936. Neuralgias and ear symptoms associated with disturbed function of the temporomandibular joint. *JAMA* 107: 252–5

Roydhouse, N. 1970. In defence of Costen's Syndrome. *J. Otolaryn. Soc. Austral.* 3: 106–14

Roydhouse, R.H. 1973. Whiplash and temporomandibular dysfunction. *Lancet* 1: 1394–5

Roydhouse, R.H., and Simonsen, B.O. 1975. Attrition of teeth. *Syesis,* in press

Sicuteri, F. 1970. Dry and wet theory in headache. *Res. Clin. Stud. Headache* 3: 159–65

Thiel, H. 1970. Zusammenhänge von Knacken und Reiben im Kiefergelenk mit anderen symptomen im Kiefer-/Gesichtsbereich. *D. Deutsch. Zahnar-zeblatt* 24: 180–8

Thomson, H. 1971. Mandibular dysfunction syndrome. *Brit. dent. J.* 130: 187–93

Timmermans, G., and Sternbach, R.A. 1974. Factors of human chronic pain: an analysis of personality of pain reaction variables. *Science* 184: 806–7

Tinbergen, N. 1974. Ethology and stress diseases. *Science* 185: 20–7

Wright, W.H. 1920. Deafness as influenced by malposition of the jaws. *J. Nat. dent. Assoc.* 7: 979–92

Yemm, R. 1969. Temporomandibular dysfunction and masseter muscle
    response to experimental stress. *Brit. dent. J.* 127: 508-10
Zobrowski, M. 1969. *People in Pain.* San Francisco: Jossey-Bass

DISCUSSION

MATTHEWS   Is it then a fair interpretation to say that these conditions do
not all fit into one definitive syndrome, that there are a large number of signs
and symptoms which tend to be treated as a common problem? If there are in
fact a number of disease states present here, would it not be profitable to undertake a survey in which the correlation between different symptoms is
looked into? If there are a number of diseases, then presumably some of these
signs and symptoms will group together.

ROYDHOUSE   I agree with you entirely. The submandibular gland swelling
and excessive salivation is a good example of an infrequently considered association. It also brings up the possibility that the autonomic nervous system is
involved. It is quite likely that there are several disorders mixed together, and
as I said before, the acceptance of trigeminal neuralgia as one part of this
group might help us resolve some of the problems associated with differentiating the real disorders.

DELLOW   The autonomic nervous system has also been implicated by Griffin
(*Med. J. Austral.* 48 [1961]: 113-16) who described a neuromyoarterial glomus adjacent to the temporomandibular joint, and suggested that compres-
sion of the glomus by the joint caused reflex autonomic changes, including
salivary changes. You have stated that 56 per cent of your patients had enlarged or painful glands. How many people without the syndrome have
enlarged or painful salivary glands?

ROYDHOUSE   I have not counted, but it would certainly be less than half the
total population.

THOMAS   I am not sure whether all your patients had muscular pain or not.
In my own experience, there always seems to be a region of muscle pain,
either in the temporalis or the masseter or the lateral pterygoid. Is that your
impression?

ROYDHOUSE   The only muscle I can clearly differentiate from head pain described by the patient, is the medial (internal) pterygoid. When the patient
states that he has regional head pain, there can be a symptomatic reaction
from many tissues in the general area and this makes a reliable diagnosis difficult. If the patient does not know that he has the muscle you are palpating,
and if it is not associated with head pain, then there is a chance for gaining
real information. The medial pterygoid seems fairly reliable in this respect.

THOMAS Berry looks for a region of spasm in a muscle, usually masseter or temporalis. I must say that one can always feel a little knot in the muscle. He uses local anaesthesia among other forms of treatment, and this does seem to relieve the muscle tension and the pain experienced by the patient. One wonders about the possibility of autonomic changes, resulting from a variety of stress inputs, as a cause of regional decreases in blood flow within the muscles. The possibility of autonomic changes being involved in the dysfunction syndrome is quite real. For example, if you extract the incisor tooth of a rodent, an enlargement of the salivary gland on the side of the extraction is produced.

ROYDHOUSE Berry's observations may well be true. This illustrates the confusion that exists. One person reports on painful muscles; another upon clicks in the temporomandibular joints. However, there does not seem to be a common aetiology, or an invariable set of signs and symptoms. There is a tendency at present to base aetiology on symptoms. The Dean of the Faculty of Dentistry in Otago used to point out that if physicians operated as dentists do, every time they saw a case of measles, they would count the number of spots and then remove them with a scalpel.

LUND How many people have you treated who had been diagnosed as having trigeminal neuralgia?

ROYDHOUSE About 8 or 9. Lindsay (1969) and Blair and Gordon (1973) both treated about 20, Kränzl and Kränzl (1973) about 80.

LUND And in the majority of cases you obtained marked improvement with relatively conservative measures?

ROYDHOUSE Yes. For example, I have adjusted occlusions, or used Tegretol, or chlordiazepoxide, or orphenadrine citrate. On occasion I have used Banthine to reduce salivary output.

LUND How accurate do you think these patients' diagnoses were?

ROYDHOUSE They had been diagnosed by neurosurgeons and neurologists. The signs and symptoms included paroxysmal pain limited to maxillary or mandibular divisions of the trigeminal nerve and trigger zones excited by light tactile stimulation, including one patient who could produce an attack by using lipstick. Most patients responded in part to treatment with Tegretol, or Dilantin sodium.

SESSLE I think my acceptance of what you are saying may be complicated by my preconceived ideas of what constitutes trigeminal neuralgia and temporomandibular joint dysfunction syndrome. The former always seemed to me to have a definite set of signs and symptoms, one of the most distinct being that only a very light tactile stimulus triggers an attack, particularly from the perioral region. Now my interpretation of what constitutes mandibular dysfunction does not include the presence of trigger zones of this kind and of this location. In passing, since Tegretol (carbamazepine) has been mentioned, we (B.J. Sessle and L.F. Greenwood, *J. dent. Res.* 54B [1975]: 201B–6B) have been carrying out studies of its mode of action. This drug, that is used so extensively to relieve trigeminal neuralgia, depresses the sensitivity of neurones in the brain stem to trigeminal sensory input. Therefore any effects resulting from afferent activity in muscle, face, teeth, etc. might be markedly reduced by this mechanism. One could give muscle spasm as an example.

DUBNER   I do not know whether we can destroy these clinical separations, as they are all we have. I agree with you, Dr Roydhouse, about aetiology – we have very little knowledge of the causes of these conditions. However, aetiology is different from signs and symptoms. We can begin to catalogue these, and set up some sort of terminology in which we can say that a given group of signs and symptoms occurring together allows us to call the phenomenon say trigeminal neuralgia, or mandibular dysfunction syndrome. If we destroy the separations, then we may end up with no way of separating out various components of the diseases.

ROYDHOUSE   One has to be careful. One of the curses of categorizing things is the assumption, prior to the event, that you know what the categories are. It is very difficult, for example, to define precisely what the myofascial pain dysfunction syndrome is. It seems to be a totally dental term, and does not seem to be present in the minds of people associated with muscle contraction headaches. I am not against cataloging signs and symptoms, in fact I would enthusiastically endorse Berry's statement that we have to catalogue the natural history of mandibular dysfunction. I would suspect that we have not catalogued it adequately in the past simply because we make assumptions that there is a difference between severe temporomandibular dysfunction and trigeminal neuralgia.

DUBNER   But you make the separation yourself because you treat some patients one way, and some another.

ROYDHOUSE   There are two ways in which one must operate. One must analyse and synthesize on the one hand, and treat people on the other. The successful treatment of patients is not necessarily directly related to an understanding of the aetiology, unfortunate though this may be. The personality of the physician may have nothing to do with the aetiology of the disorder, but it may have a lot to do with the success of the treatment.

STOREY   You have a fairly large component of accident victims in your sample. In these cases, what sort of treatment seems effective? Does occlusal equilibration work?

ROYDHOUSE   On the basis of clinical observation, it appears that if you treat the patient with the assumption that the mandible is displaced, then you seem to end up with more success than if you start in any other fashion. This displacement may be permanent in some cases, or temporary in others. In many cases one may arrive at a symptomless condition when the mandible has returned to an apparently normal relationship with the maxilla.

STOREY   Are these displacements caused by muscles?

ROYDHOUSE   I assume so. The way one recognizes the displacement is by observing that the teeth do not fit together in the way that they obviously did before. One is often helped in this by factors like wear facets.

KAWAMURA   It is often said that the mandibular dysfunction patients fall into a young and a middle-aged group. Have you been able to follow up any of your patients over a long period?

ROYDHOUSE   I cannot recognize that there are these two groups. From the survey of the literature and my own patients, it would seem that everyone has an equal opportunity to have mandibular dysfunction. My youngest patient was aged 7, and my oldest 75. I admit that two-thirds to three-quarters are female. To gather the sort of information you want, one would have to have a proper epidemiological survey. With the exception of the work of Agerberg and Carlsson (*Acta odont. scand.* 30 [1972] : 597–613), proper epidemiological methods do not appear to have been used in any survey of mandibular dysfunction.

Some considerations of synaptic organization in the trigeminal sensory nuclei of the adult cat

STEPHEN GOBEL

Two major sources of excitatory input to the cranial motor nuclei are derived from (1) reflexo-motor primary afferent axons from the cranial musculature and (2) second-order neurones located in the sensory nuclei of the trigeminal, glossopharyngeal, and vagus nerves. In attempting to understand complex reflex activity of the cranial musculature, it is essential to first consider how sensory input from these two sources is processed before it is relayed to the cranial motoneurones. This report will consider several aspects of the synaptic organization of the main sensory (MSN) and spinal trigeminal (SP V) nuclei.

The neurones which make up MSN and SP V may be divided into projection neurones, i.e. neurones whose axons leave their parent nucleus, and interneurones, i.e. neurones whose axons arborize entirely within the trigeminal nuclei. Projection neurones include trigemino-thalamic neurones (Darian-Smith and Yokota, 1966), trigemino-reticular neurones (Ramón y Cajal, 1909, Figs. 302 and 368), and neurones which project to the cranial motor nuclei (Ramón y Cajal, 1909, Figs. 302 and 311). Interneurones include Golgi type II neurones whose axons arborize in the general vicinity of their dendritic trees, e.g., the neurones of the substantia gelatinosa layer of nucleus caudalis. SP V also contains interneurones whose axons project for considerable distances within the nucleus (Gobel and Purvis, 1972). The output of the trigeminal sensory nuclei to the cranial motor nuclei is largely determined by synaptic interactions between trigeminal primary afferent axons, interneurones, and the projection neurones.

With the exceptions of the marginal layer of nucleus caudalis and the interstitial nucleus, synaptic transfers between primary trigeminal afferent axons and neurones of the trigeminal sensory nuclei take place in structures called glomeruli. The simplest glomerulus is made up of three kinds of neuronal processes (Fig. 1). A large axonal ending (C) with large spherical synaptic vesicles is surrounded by several dendritic processes of different sizes (D) and by smaller axonal endings (P) with smaller mixed spherical and flattened vesicles

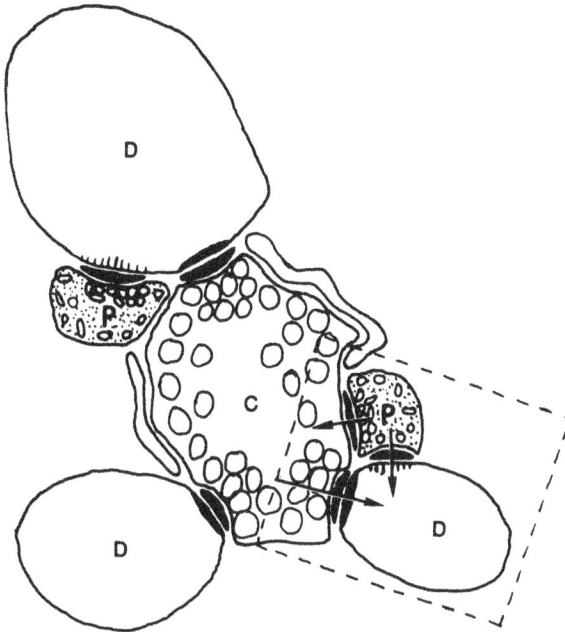

FIGURE 1   A typical MSN glomerulus consists of a trigeminal nerve ending (C), dendrites (D), and small axonal endings with small synaptic vesicles (P). The three processes are linked together by three synapses which form the basis of integrative structural units (dashed rectangle).

(Gobel and Dubner, 1969). Degeneration studies following trigeminal nerve rhizotomy have shown that the C axonal endings in MSN (Gobel, 1971) and SP V (Westrum and Black, 1971) glomeruli are derived from trigeminal primary afferent axons. The three neuronal processes are linked together by three kinds of synapses (Fig. 1): the C axon forms asymmetric (Gray's type I) synapses on the dendrites and the P axonal endings form intermediate axodendritic synapses on the dendrites and symmetrical (Gray's type II) axoaxonic synapses on the C axon.

Glomeruli may be divided into smaller structural units based on these three synapses (Fig. 1, dashed rectangle). It is within these structural units that information transmitted by primary afferent axons is modified, probably by inhibitory mechanisms, through the axodendritic and axoaxonic synapses of the P ending before being relayed out of the trigeminal nuclei.

Such integrative mechanisms may be considered more clearly when the source of the P axons of the trigeminal glomeruli is considered. The SP V nucleus contains an extensive plexus of small bundles of axons (the deep bun-

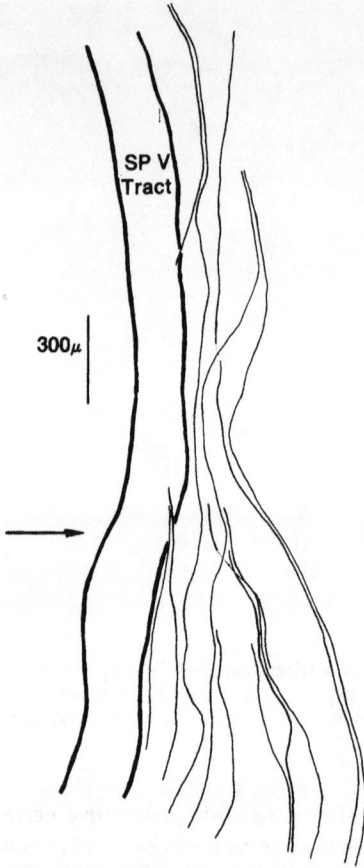

FIGURE 2 Camera lucida drawing made from a horizontal section of a Golgi preparation through nucleus oralis (above arrow) and nucleus interpolaris (below arrow). Each thin line has been traced down the centre of a deep bundle and illustrates the plexus-like nature of the deep bundles (Reproduced, with permission, from *Brain Res.* 48 [1972]: 27–44).

dles) which run longitudinally through SP V (Fig. 2). Each bundle contains about a thousand axons, about half of which are unmyelinated (Gobel and Purvis, 1972, Fig. 12). Eighty to ninety per cent of the myelinated axons are less than 1.5μ in diameter (Gobel and Purvis, 1972, Fig. 11). Observations made from Golgi studies (Gobel and Purvis, 1972) and degeneration studies (Gobel, 1971) reveal that many of the axons in the deep bundles are derived from neurones of SP V, while only a few primary trigeminal axons run in the deep bundles. Axons of SP V neurones on entering the deep bundles may either ascend or descend for considerable distances in SP V and in their course

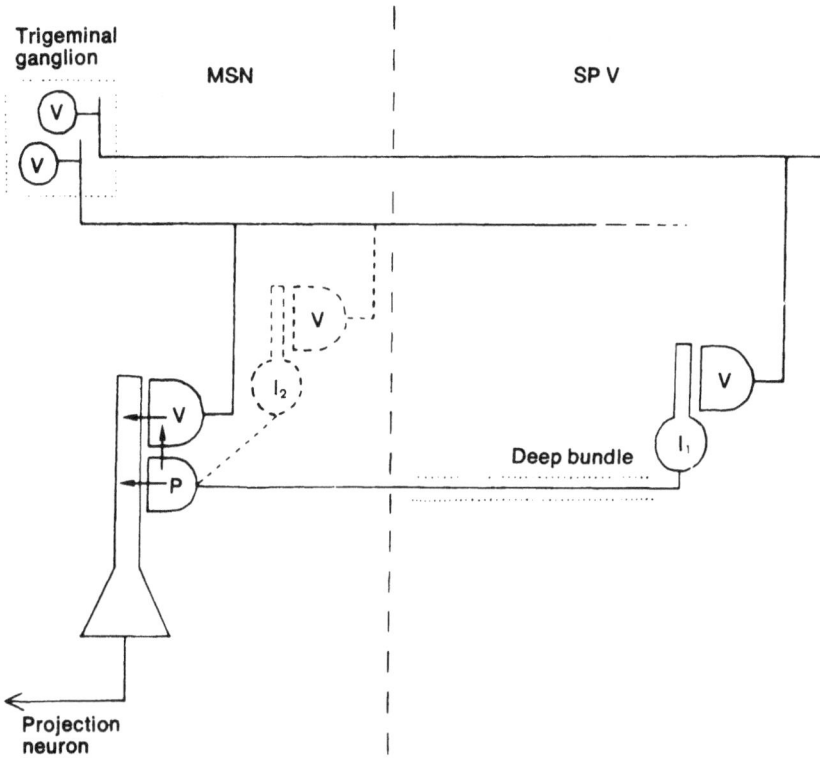

FIGURE 3 Summary of the major circuits involving trigeminal (V) nerve endings in the MSN and SP V nuclei. Axonal endings (P) of interneurones (I) form axoaxonic synapses on V nerve endings and axodendritic synapses on projection neurone dendrites.

emit widely spaced collaterals. These collaterals possess fine boutons *en passant* and a few fine end boutons (Gobel and Purvis, 1972, Figs. 15-19) which correlate closely with the size and shape of the P axonal endings seen in the glomeruli.

If SP V is transected at the level of the obex, some degenerating P axonal endings can be found in glomeruli in parts of SP V rostral to the site of transection (Gobel, 1971, Figs. 26 and 27). These observations are summarized in Figure 3 and suggest that the projection neurones of MSN and SP V are involved in the following synaptic circuits. Primary trigeminal axons form excitatory axodendritic synapses on the dendrites of a projection neurone, in MSN for example, and on the dendrites of interneurones (Fig. 3, I_1 and I_2). Along with activation of the projection neurone, inhibitory interneurones are also activated. The latter in turn exert an inhibitory effect on the projection neurone postsynaptically through axodendritic synapses and presynaptically through axoaxonic synapses. Interneurones may send their axons into the deep bundles to reach projection neurones some distance away (Fig. 3, I_1). In addition, interneurones in the immediate vicinity of the projection neurone (Fig. 3, I_2) would also be involved in these circuits. These synaptic circuits between primary trigeminal axonal endings, projection neurones and inhibitory interneurones are probably involved in shaping inhibitory surrounds and integrating inputs from neighbouring peripheral receptive fields on the second-order neurones.

The substantia gelatinosa (SG) layer of the lower end of SP V, i.e. nucleus caudalis, receives a prolific trigeminal primary input (Ramón y Cajal, 1909; Kerr, 1970, 1971; Gobel, 1971, 1974a). Based on clinical experience with trigeminal tractotomy procedures associated with trigeminal neuralgia (Sjöqvist, 1938; Kunc, 1970) and the presence of neurones in nucleus caudalis which respond exclusively to nociceptive stimuli (Mosso and Kruger, 1973), this primary trigeminal input to SG would appear to be essential to the perception and appreciation of oro-facial pain. The synaptic connections in the SG layer between primary afferent axons, projection neurones and interneurones are more complex than in other sites in MSN and SP V (Fig. 4). This is due in part to the presence of three morphologically distinct neuronal cell types in the SG layer (Gobel, 1974b). The axonal and dendritic morphology of these SG neurones suggest that they all function as Golgi type II inhibitory interneurones. The axons of these three SG neurones do not project out of SP V.

Projection neurones of nucleus caudalis are located in the magnocellular layer (Gordon et al., 1961; Darian-Smith and Yokota, 1966) and possibly also in the marginal layer. Many neurones in these layers send their dendrites into the SG layer (Gobel, 1974b) where they receive part of their trigeminal primary input in the SG glomeruli and where they come under the influence of the SG interneurones. In SG glomeruli (Fig. 4) a trigeminal primary axonal ending (C), identified as such in degeneration studies (Gobel, 1974a, Fig. 23), forms asymmetrical axodendritic synapses on two kinds of dendritic spines (1 and 2) and on dendritic shafts (D). These dendritic elements are in turn linked together by two kinds of dendrodendritic synapses. Type 2 spines containing large synaptic vesicles form intermediate dendrodendritic synapses on type 1 spines, while dendritic shafts containing clusters of small synaptic vesicles form symmetrical dendrodendritic synapses among themselves and on type 1 spines. P axons form axoaxonic synapses on trigeminal primary axonal endings (P → C) and axodendritic synapses (P → 1 and P → D) as they do in the integrative structural units of the simpler trigeminal glomeruli (Fig. 1).

The internal synaptic circuitry of the SG glomeruli is arranged as follows. Trigeminal nerve endings simultaneously activate the dendrites of projection

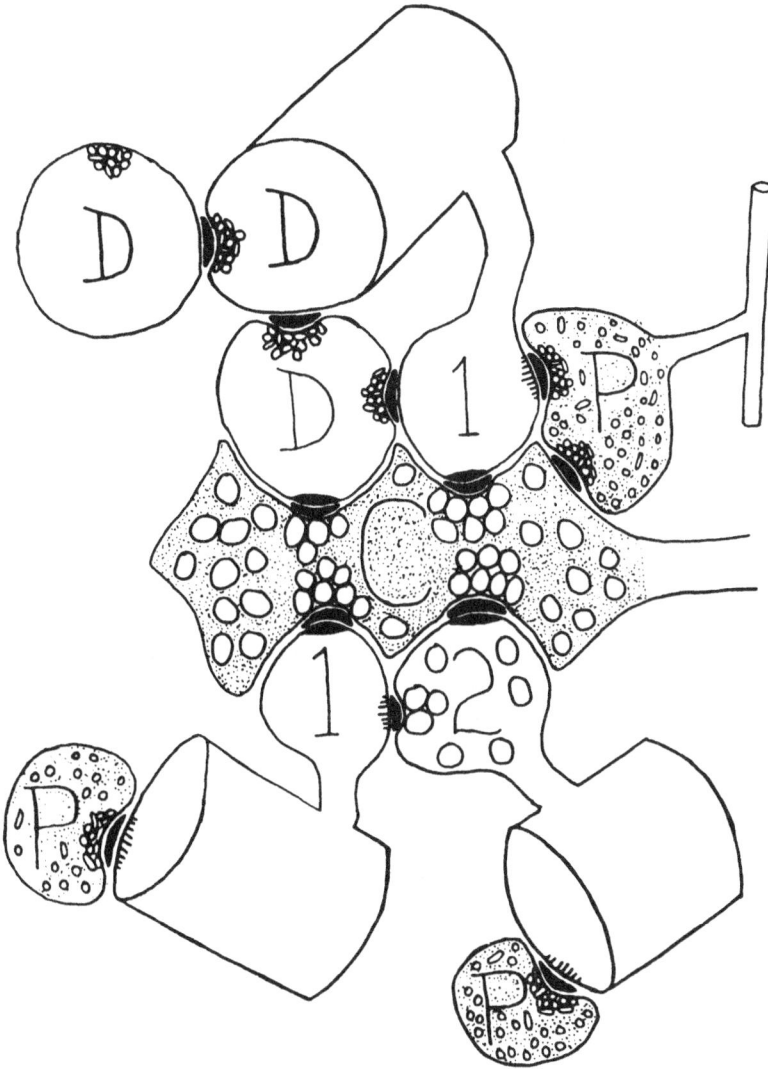

FIGURE 4 Summary of the neuronal constituents of the glomeruli of the SG layer of nucleus caudalis and their synaptic connections (Reproduced, with permission, from *J. Neurocytol.* 3 [1974] : 219–43).

neurones and interneurones largely through their dendritic spines. Projection neurones, whose cell bodies are located in either the marginal or magnocellular layers, may also excite SG interneurones through an excitatory dendro-dendritic synapse (type 2 spine → type 1 spine). Activation of the interneurone, in turn, would inhibit transmission in the afferent axon-projection neurone circuit through its axoaxonic synapses (P → C) and possibly through axodendritic synapses (P → D). Inhibitory connections between one or more morphological types of SG interneurones are effected through the dendrodendritic synapses between vesicle-containing dendritic shafts, between dendritic shafts and type 1 spines, and possibly also between axodendritic synapses. A broader discussion of these circuits is presented elsewhere (Gobel, 1974a).

CONCLUSIONS

Unlike stretch reflexes of the cranial musculature which usually involve direct synaptic contact between the sensory cells and motoneurones, e.g., trigeminal mesencephalic neurone → trigeminal motoneurone, reflexes and cranial motor activity involving the sensory root of the trigeminal nerve are more complex and involve three or more neurones. Many of the neurones of MSN and SP V project to the cranial motor nuclei where they effect the transfer of information from primary trigeminal axons to cranial motoneurones. Part of this process involves the activation of the interneurones in MSN and SP V. These neurones in turn feed back into fifth nerve-projection neurone circuits where, based on morphological criteria, they are considered to exert an inhibitory effect through axoaxonic synapses on the trigeminal nerve endings and axodendritic synapses on the projection neurones. Some of the most complex processing of V nerve input takes place in the glomeruli of the SG layer. In these glomeruli, trigeminal nerve axons thought to be related to pain and temperature sensations appear to interact with three different interneurones before being relayed out of SP V. These studies indicate that, in addition to considering synaptic events on the cranial motoneurone surface, it is equally important to consider the synaptic events in the cranial sensory nuclei if we are to delineate accurately the neural pathways underlying the complex reflexes which form the basis of mastication and swallowing.

REFERENCES

Darian-Smith, I., and Yokota, T. 1966. Corticofugal effects on different neuron types within the cat's brain stem activated by tactile stimulation of the face. *J. Neurophysiol.* 29: 185–206
Gobel, S. 1971. Structural organization in the main sensory trigeminal nucleus. In R. Dubner and Y. Kawamura (eds.), *Oral-Facial Sensory and Motor Mechanisms.* New York: Appleton-Century-Crofts

- 1974a. Synaptic organization of the substantia gelatinosa glomeruli in the spinal trigeminal nucleus. *J. Neurocytol.* 3: 219-43
- 1974b. Identification of the neurons which contribute to the neuropil of the substantia gelatinosa layer of the spinal trigeminal nucleus in the adult cat. A Golgi study. *Anat. Rec.* 178: 497

Gobel, S., and Dubner, R. 1969. Fine structural studies of the main sensory trigeminal nucleus in the cat and rat. *J. comp. Neurol.* 137: 459-93

Gobel, S., and Purvis, M.B. 1972. Anatomical studies of the organization of the spinal V nucleus: The deep bundles and the spinal V tract. *Brain Res.* 48: 27-44

Gordon, G., Landgren, S., and Seed, W.A. 1961. The functional characteristics of single cells in the caudal part of the spinal nucleus of the trigeminal nerve of the cat. *J. Physiol. (Lond.)* 158: 544-59

Kerr, F.W.L. 1970. The organization of primary afferents in the subnucleus caudalis of the trigeminal: a light and electron microscopic study of degeneration. *Brain Res.* 23: 147-65

- 1971. Electron microscopic observations on primary deafferentation of subnucleus caudalis of the trigeminal nerve. In R. Dubner and Y. Kawamura (eds.), *Oral-Facial Sensory and Motor Mechanisms.* New York: Appleton-Century-Crofts

Kunc, Z. 1970. Significant factors pertaining to the results of trigeminal tractotomy. In R. Hassler and A.E. Walker (eds.), *Trigeminal Neuralgia: Pathogenesis and Pathophysiology.* Philadelphia: Saunders

Mosso, J.A., and Kruger, L. 1973. Receptor categories represented in spinal trigeminal nucleus caudalis. *J. Neurophysiol.* 36: 472-88

Ramón y Cajal, S. 1909. *Histologie du Système Nerveux de l'Homme et des Vertébrés.* Vol. 1. Madrid: Instituto Ramón y Cajal (1952 Reprint)

Sjöqvist, O. 1938. Studies of pain conduction in the trigeminal nerve. A contribution to the surgical treatment of facial pain. *Acta Psychiatrica et Neurologica Scandinavica. Suppl.* 17: 1-139

Westrum, L.E., and Black, R.G. 1971. Fine structural aspects of the synaptic organization of the spinal trigeminal nucleus (pars interpolaris) of the cat. *Brain Res.* 25: 265-88

DISCUSSION

DUBNER I thought we could begin this discussion by considering the delayed inhibition seen in the jaw-elevator muscles, and how specific this delayed inhibition might be for nociceptive information.

GOLDBERG I do not think you can be very firm about it being solely related to noxious inputs. One can speculate that this inhibition is involved with motor mechanisms; it is not necessary to stimulate electrically high-threshold fibres in order to evoke it.

LUND I am concerned that when we study, for example, a monosynaptic reflex, or look at our inhibitory patterns in the elevator muscles, what we see may be strongly influenced by the methods we use to evoke the response. If one gives a short-duration electrical shock, then what we may be looking at is transmission through the main input line only with very little modification. If we deliver a train of impulses, or a natural stimulus, we may obtain a very different output because we are now, in time, seeing more pre and postsynaptic modification of the incoming information. I think this sort of thing is a source of much confusion.

GOLDBERG Dr Gobel, is there any organization of the arborizations in the nucleus oralis? Are axoaxonic synapses only found on fifth nerve terminals and are they found near the boutons?

GOBEL With respect to the collaterals, we do not have the answer to that. I have followed a few collaterals in the new-born rat, and there does seem to be a spatial distribution of fifth nerve endings. When we work out the specifics, I think we will find things very nicely organized. The peripheral (P) endings synapse only on fifth nerve *terminals*. I should also add that we find P endings out on dendritic shafts and on cell bodies outside the glomeruli.

With respect to the morphology of fifth nerve endings in the substantia layer, there is a morphological difference. The shapes of the terminals are different. In the trigeminal main sensory nucleus and spinal nucleus they tend to be bulbous, whereas in the substantia layer of caudalis they are more elongated and their borders are scalloped. Also, there is a difference in inherent electron density. The endings in the substantia layer are darker. This difference is not a procedural artefact. I think this is an important point, because Ramón y Cajal (1909) found in his methylene blue preparations of primary cell bodies in the trigeminal ganglion, that he could divide them into large, pale cell bodies and smaller, dark cell bodies. Other studies have confirmed this at an electron microscopic level (R. Peach. *J. Neurocytol.* 1 [1972]: 151-60). If you disregard organelles and just compare the densities of the cytoplasm in the small dark cells and in the axoplasm of the substantia fifth nerve endings, they are very similar. The other piece of circumstantial evidence which leads me to believe that the substantia endings are the endings of those small, dark cells is that the small cells have a very high acid phosphatase content. The fifth nerve endings also have this, but only in the substantia layer (A. Rustioni et al., *Brain Res.* 32 [1971]: 45-52). Thus it is beginning to appear that we have a basis for predicting that the small, trigeminal neurones may be going to a specific place in the trigeminal nucleus.

LUND Have you tried to type the synaptic vesicles?

GOBEL Yes, the synaptic vesicles in the fifth nerve endings are large spheres or ellipsoids. If you measure their short diameters they are about 400 Å. If you define a flattened vesicle as a vesicle whose long diameter exceeds its short diameter by a factor of 2, then flattened vesicles comprise less than 1 per cent of the synaptic vesicles of the endings. On the other hand, the vesicles in the P ending are about 100 Å narrower, and contain a higher number of flattened vesicles, anywhere from 3 to 29 per cent. The same kind of breakdown occurs in the two dendrites with synaptic vesicles. I think all of our experience with electron microscopical studies in sensory systems leads to the conclusion that endings with small vesicles are inhibitory. All primary afferent endings have large vesicles and are excitatory and the interneurones have small vesicles and are inhibitory.

DUBNER By these anatomical criteria then, the only interneurones that you have identified are inhibitory interneurones. Would you like to speculate how caudalis can have a facilitatory effect on the more rostral parts of the trigeminal brain stem complex if the only intranuclear connections are via inhibitory interneurones?

GOBEL I want to emphasize that I have looked at two locations, the main sensory nucleus and the substantia layer of caudalis and my remarks are concerned with these locations. I have not looked at the rest of the trigeminal spinal nucleus and this area is quite extensive. The type II spine may or may not belong to an interneurone. I have not determined this yet. With respect to the facilitatory effect of caudalis, I envision two kinds of intrinsic connections along the length of the trigeminal spinal nucleus. We have long-distance connections: for example, some neurones send their axons from caudalis up to oralis in the deep bundles or the spinal tract, and then we have others which are shorter, i.e. classical Golgi type II neurones whose axons are restricted to the immediate area of their dendritic arbors. What could be happening in transecting or cooling caudalis is that only part of this complex of interneurones is cut off, i.e. the long-distance connections. Perhaps this releases Golgi type II neurones in the vicinity of the projection neurone which is being monitored in rostral parts of the trigeminal nuclear complex. Dr Sessle, you have also postulated inhibitory effects from caudalis, haven't you?

SESSLE We have never postulated that the facilitatory effect we have observed is due to one neurone in caudalis projecting all the way to the main sensory nucleus (B.J. Sessle and L.F. Greenwood, *Brain Res.* 67 [1974]: 330-3; and *J. dent. Res.* 54 [1975]: 201B-6B). But we would not disagree with what you have postulated. In blocking caudalis, we are looking at the overall influence of caudalis which seems to be primarily facilitatory, but there is evidence of an inhibitory influence as well, and this is indicated also by others (D. Denny-Brown and N. Yanagisawa, *Brain* 96 [1973]: 783-814). You were wondering what neurone(s) might be involved in the projection. Only 40 per cent of the neurones in caudalis project to the thalamus (e.g. M.J. Rowe and B.J. Sessle, *Brain Res.* 42 [1972]: 367-84), but others may pass to the motor nuclei, and many project to the reticular formation. So again there is a lot of room for speculating that these could be the pathways that are involved in the effects of caudalis on sensory transmission and also on reflex function.

GOBEL There are also a lot of axons within the spinal tract which survive after fifth nerve rhizotomy and most of these belong to the intrinsic neurones of the trigeminal nuclei. The number of surviving axons outnumbers the number of degenerating axons by probably 10 to 1, and this assessment is only based on myelinated axons.

SESSLE That in itself is certainly a remarkable observation, and yet you said, I think, that with respect to the input to the substantia gelatinosa, the central axons are derived only from trigeminal nerve fibres. Is that correct?

GOBEL Yes. My work is based upon the first two rostral millimetres of caudalis only. The central endings in the substantia layer are trigeminal primary afferents. What the extent of overlap between the trigeminal nerve, cranial nerves VII, IX, and X and the upper cervical nerves is at any particular point, remains to be determined (see below).

SESSLE What about the origin of P axons?

GOBEL After trigeminal rhizotomy, the P endings do not degenerate. The unmyelinated axons do not degenerate. I think that the bulk of the unmyelinated axons and P endings in the substantia layer are derived from the axons of the neurones that make up that layer.

STOREY I wonder if you could comment on the similarities between the substantia layer of the trigeminal nucleus and that of the spinal cord.

GOBEL There appear to be basic similarities in terms of the morphology of the glomeruli, the dark primary afferent endings, and the presence of axoaxonic synapses on the primary afferent axons. Detailed comparisons of synaptic circuitry are not possible at this time.

HANNAM Would you comment on the relationship between the trigeminal system and C1, C2, and C3 segments of the spinal cord? This area has strong clinical significance, yet from a neurophysiological aspect, very little study seems to have been conducted. We know that there are anatomical connections between dorsal root afferents from the upper three cervical segments and the trigeminal spinal nucleus, and we also know that mandibular dysfunction symptoms not infrequently include soreness in the trapezius and sterno-mastoid muscles.

GOBEL   There are a few things we can say concerning the primary afferent input to the substantia layer in caudalis and in the upper cervical cord. I think it is accepted now that there are some fifth nerve axons that go down to C2 and C3. In fact, the results of Rustioni et al. (1971) would suggest that the ophthalmic division does not terminate in the substantia layer in caudalis, but that it terminates at C1 and C2. They would also suggest that those parts of cranial nerves VII, IX and X that travel in the spinal tract do not terminate in caudalis, but in the substantia layer of the upper cervical segments (A. Rustioni et al., *Brain Res.* 37 [1972]: 137-40). This area should be looked at thoroughly with the electron miscroscope.

SESSLE   Moreover, no physiological study has been made for instance of the cervical, glossopharyngeal, or laryngeal input to this area. We do not know how it is interacting here with the trigeminal input, although such interactions do occur elsewhere, such as the main sensory and solitary tract nuclei (e.g. B.J. Sessle, *Brain Res.* 53 [1973]: 319-31).

Pain, brain stem mechanisms, and motor function

L.F. GREENWOOD AND B.J. SESSLE

The effects of pain on motor function in the oral-facial area are not easy to investigate. Production of a pure pain stimulus is difficult, and, while it is generally considered that bipolar electrical stimulation of the tooth pulp gives rise only to pain in man (e.g. Anderson, Hannam, and Matthews, 1970), the sensation produced at threshold levels of stimulation is not always described as painful (Mumford, 1965; Hannam, Siu, and Tom, 1974). Conversely, a painful stimulus produces many effects apart from the sensory experience. In the trigeminal area these include (i) referral of pain to deep structures, especially muscles and the temporomandibular joint (TMJ), (ii) jaw, facial, and tongue muscle reflexes, (iii) changes in respiratory and autonomic activities, and (iv) behavioural changes such as grimacing. Further problems are posed by the complex inter-relationships between facial, tongue, laryngeal, pharyngeal, and jaw muscles, and by the use of animals; for instance, in the cat the digastric is a significant jaw-opening muscle (e.g. Thexton, 1973) whereas in man its importance is still controversial (Munro, 1972; Yemm, 1972). There is evidence too that neospinothalamic pathways concerned with pain are different in man and non-primates (for review see Mehler, 1969).

These problems may account for the small amount of physiological information we have linking pain and oral-facial muscle function. Such evidence as we have is almost entirely on jaw muscles, with little or nothing on tongue, facial, laryngeal, or pharyngeal musculature, and even this evidence appears to be paradoxical. High-intensity oral-facial stimulation almost invariably produces jaw opening in the experimental situation, with digastric activation and masseter inhibition (e.g. Thexton, 1973), while painful conditions of the trigeminal region, the temporomandibular joint pain dysfunction syndrome for example, are associated with trismus, that is, activation of the jaw-closing muscles.

Sherrington's (1917) early work with decerebrate cats described only a jaw-opening movement, with stimulation of the teeth, palate, or gingiva, but later workers describe both digastric excitation and masseter inhibition. The reflex can be evoked by stimulation of many oral-facial sites, although there is no evidence of a short-latency input from muscle spindles to digastric motoneurones (Kidokoro et al., 1968; and see Table 1: lack of MES V input). The large number of sites from which the reflex can be evoked is reflected in the wide variety of inputs to digastric motoneurones revealed by our recent micro-electrode study of single trigeminal motoneurones in anaesthetized and decerebrate cats (see Fig. 1 and Table 1). Experimental details, and the identification of the alpha and gamma motoneurones listed in Table 1 are described briefly elsewhere (Greenwood and Sessle, 1973); the responses of a gamma motoneurone are shown in Figure 1. There were also significant facilitatory effects, especially with tooth tapping or tooth pulp stimulation (Table 2), but for most conditioning stimuli the early facilitation was followed by inhibition. Conditioning effects have also been demonstrated from vagal afferents (Chase, Torii, and Nakamura, 1970), and limb nerves (e.g. Kubota, Kidokoro, and Suzuki, 1968).

Work in man has concentrated largely on the masseter inhibition, since in this case jaw opening can occur without digastric activation (Yemm, 1972). Two phases of inhibition occur; an early one which is evoked even with innocuous stimuli, and a later one which seems to require a high-intensity or painful stimulus (see Yu, Schmitt, and Sessle, 1973 for review).

Even though the jaw-opening reflex is classically considered as a protective reflex, elicited only by high-intensity stimulation, it can be evoked by quite small stimuli. For instance Kidokoro et al. (1968) evoked it with 1.25 times threshold stimulation of the inferior dental nerve (IDN), Schmitt, Yu, and Sessle (1973) with threshold superior laryngeal nerve (SLN) stimulation, Sessle and Greenwood (unpublished observations) with light mechanical stimulation of a tooth and with infra-orbital nerve (IO) stimulation equal to that required for threshold facial muscle activation (contrary to Keller, Vyklicky, and Sykova, 1972), and Mahan and Anderson (1970) and Reid (1972) with tooth pulp stimulation which appeared to be non-painful in cats. These examples might indicate that the reflex is not necessarily only protective in function, since it can be elicited by small, presumably non-painful stimuli, although the low-intensity electrical stimuli used in nearly all of these studies do not duplicate physiological stimulation.

TABLE 1 Excitatory inputs to trigeminal motoneurones. Horizontal rows denote type of motoneurone, and vertical columns denote the number of motoneurones having an input and tested, and where applicable the mean latency (LAT) for excitation ± standard error in milliseconds (msec). M = masseter, T = temporalis, D = digastric, ANTI = antidromic, MES V = trigeminal mesencephalic nucleus, TT = tooth tap, TP = tooth pulp, IO = infraorbital nerve, IX = glossopharyngeal nerve, SLN = superior laryngeal nerve, FP = forepaw.

	ANTI	LAT (msec)	MES V	LAT (msec)	TT	LAT (msec)	TP	LAT (msec)
M_a	122	0.98 ± 0.02	39/44	0.92 ± 0.02	30/48	6.16 ± 0.28	0/37	
M_γ	34	1.52 ± 0.03	8/13	1.61 ± 0.16	9/15	6.71 ± 0.63	0/9	
T_a	38	1.06 ± 0.04	13/18	0.92 ± 0.03	11/18	8.44 ± 0.90	0/12	
T_γ	10	1.70 ± 0.04	9/9	1.31 ± 0.07	6/6	8.58 ± 0.54	0/3	
D	58	1.24 ± 0.06	0/40		16/33	8.38 ± 0.63	9/29	6.35 ± 0.98

	IO	LAT (msec)	IX	LAT (msec)	SLN	LAT (msec)	FP	LAT (msec)
M_a	0/57		2/56	7.0	0/56		1/36	20.0
M_γ	2/12	8.0	0/13		0/13		0/9	
T_a	2/14	18.0	2/13	13.0	2/14	18.0	0/6	
T_γ	1/3	6.0	1/3	8.0	0/2		0	
D	12/36	6.35 ± 0.52	15/38	8.86 ± 0.50	9/38	8.75 ± 0.68	0/17	

TABLE 2 Conditioning of trigeminal motoneurones. Horizontal rows denote type of motoneurone, vertical columns denote conditioning stimulus and number of motoneurones tested, and of these the number facilitated (↑), depressed or inhibited (↓) or unaffected (x). Facilitatory effects were generally short lasting (<60 msec), while many inhibitory effects lasted longer than 100 msec and were sometimes preceded by an early facilitation. Abbreviations as for Table 1

	TT	↑	↓	x	TP	↑	↓	x	IO	↑	↓	x
Ma	42	5	25	12	16	1	5	10	17	3	8	6
Mγ	15	1	13	1	6	0	3	3	8	0	5	3
Ta	13	4	8	1	4	0	3	1	6	0	3	3
Tγ	4	1	3	0	3	0	2	1	1	0	1	0
D	19	14	2	3	12	9	0	3	7	3	2	2

	IX	↑	↓	x	SLN	↑	↓	x	FP	↑	↓	x
Ma	28	8	7	13	28	3	6	19	5	0	0	5
Mγ	9	0	5	4	10	0	4	6	4	0	1	3
Ta	9	1	5	3	11	1	5	5	3	0	2	1
Tγ	2	0	1	1	2	0	0	2	0			
D	15	9	3	3	12	6	3	3	6	1	0	5

	D	↑	↓	x	T	↑	↓	x	M	↑	↓	x
Ma	10	0	4	6	11	2	5	4	9	0	9	0
Mγ	3	0	0	3	3	0	2	1	6	0	6	0
Ta	4	1	0	3	4	0	3	1	8	0	7	1
Tγ	0				0				0			
D	1	0	0	1	4	0	1	3	5	1	1	3

Brain stem pathways

Sumino (1971) reported that in the adult cat the digastric reflex evoked by IDN stimulation is disynaptic, with the interneurone in trigeminal nucleus oralis or interpolaris. Nucleus caudalis also appears to influence the reflex since Riblet and Mitchell (1972) showed that the inhibitory effect of morphine on the digastric reflex evoked by tooth pulp stimulation was reduced by section of the trigeminal sensory nucleus and tract at the obex. We have shown that cold block of caudalis produces reversible depression of digastric and facial reflexes evoked by IO, tooth pulp, and tooth tap stimuli (Sessle and Greenwood, unpublished observations), although it does not affect the response of either trigeminal primary afferent fibres or the antidromic response to trigeminal motoneurones (Sessle and Greenwood, 1975). The mechanism of this inhibition is not known, but possibly entails either a pre or postsynaptic inhibition of a second-order cell in the rostral trigeminal sensory nuclei by re-

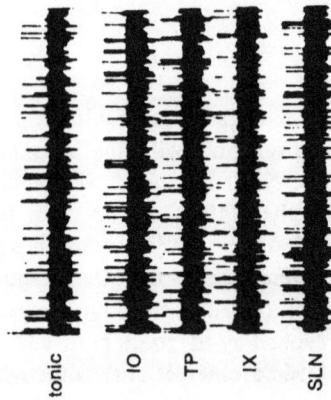

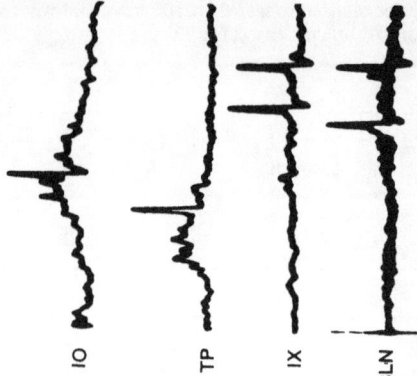

FIGURE 1 Masseter motoneurones receive few inputs from peripheral sites compared with digastric motoneurones. On the left are shown five superimposed antidromic responses of a masseter gamma motoneurone (calibration: 0.2 mV; 1 msec) and records (calibration: 20 msec) showing its spontaneous activity and that following electrical stimulation of the infraorbital nerve (IO), canine tooth pulp (TP), glossopharyngeal nerve (IX), and superior laryngeal nerve (SLN). A similar set of records are shown on the right for a digastric motoneurone which was not spontaneously active (calibration: 0.2 mV; 1 msec, antidromic responses; 2 msec other responses). Note that the digastric motoneurone was activated by all the stimuli, while the masseter motoneurone was activated by none of them. The gamma motoneurone exhibited a typically long-latency, high-threshold response to antidromic stimulation, lack of monosynaptic excitation from the trigeminal mesencephalic nucleus, and discharged tonically even with the jaw closed.

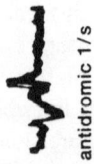

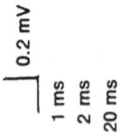

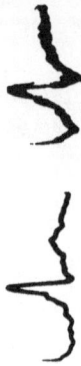

moval of a tonic facilitatory effect exerted by nucleus caudalis. There is anatomical and physiological evidence for both ascending and descending intranuclear connections which could furnish the pathway for both pre and postsynaptic modulation of the rostral sensory cells by caudalis, as discussed in
Gobel's presentation.

JAW-CLOSING REFLEX

The jaw-opening reflex demonstrates one response of the oral-facial musculature to a painful stimulus, but does not provide a link between pain and spasm
of the jaw-closing muscles. This symposium has already covered some of the
influences which can activate or facilitate jaw-closing muscles, but these are
few and weak compared with those which affect digastric motoneurones under similar experimental conditions. Tables 1 and 2 summarize some of our
results from single jaw-closing motoneurones. It is evident that with the exception of tooth tapping there is little or no short-latency excitatory input to
jaw-closing motoneurones, and that the predominant conditioning effect on
both alpha and gamma motoneurones from all the sites tested is an inhibition,
sometimes preceded by an early facilitation. Again with the exception of
those effects of tooth tapping, the conditioning effects were not as common
as those on digastric motoneurones.

We have little or no evidence on the effects of high-threshold muscle afferent fibres on motoneurones. Nakamura and his colleagues (1973) demonstrated that stimulation of masseteric Group II afferents, arising possibly from
non-spindle sources such as Pacinian corpuscles and free nerve endings, produces an early facilitation followed by a long-lasting, two-phased inhibition in
masseter motoneurones and in the masseteric reflex. In an earlier paper (1971)
they showed that high-threshold masseteric afferents had only inhibitory
effects on the masseter motoneurones and reflex. Electrical stimulation of the
tooth pulp, the nearest approximation to a pure pain stimulus in our experiments, showed little evidence of any excitatory effect on masseter or temporalis motoneurones, and its conditioning effects were almost entirely inhibitory (Tables 1 and 2). This contrasts with the elicitation of facial and tongue
reflexes by high-intensity stimulation of oral-facial afferent fibres (for review,
see Sessle and Kenny, 1973). One reason for this apparent lack of excitatory
input to jaw-closing motoneurones is masking by the concomitant inhibitory
effects of the same stimuli. Facilitation may be uncovered by the use of
strychnine (Kidokoro et al., 1968; Sumino, 1971).

Another reason for the apparent lack may be that the stimulus characteristics have not been appropriate; most workers have used electrical stimulation,
but even if a more physiological mechanical form of stimulus is employed,
the strength and duration (Achari and Thexton, 1974) or direction (Funa-

koshi and Amano, 1974) of effective stimuli may be very limited. In the case of the central inputs and conditioning effects on trigeminal motoneurones, it may be that the more widespread use of non-anaesthetized preparations will reveal more effects and enhance our knowledge of the influence of the sleep state of the animal on them. This in turn may help to explain phenomena such as bruxism and the TMJ pain-dysfunction syndrome(s).

Brain stem pathways

In any discussion of pain in the trigeminal region, nucleus caudalis is inevitably implicated. In the previous paper Gobel has discussed some of its intra- and extra-nuclear ramifications and reviewed the anatomical literature. It receives small afferent fibres from a variety of sources (see Kerr, 1972 for review), but as yet we do not know if it receives small muscle afferents from the trigeminal region, and descriptions of primary nociceptor relays in the nucleus (Greenwood, 1973; Mosso and Kruger, 1973) were not adequately confirmed by histological evidence or their central projections determined. The early facilitation and late inhibition of the masseteric reflex and the associated changes in membrane potential of masseter motoneurones are either reduced or abolished by section of the trigeminal spinal nucleus at or near the obex (e.g. Sumino, 1971; Nakamura et al., 1973). It is possible that this section directly cuts off a relay neurone in the nucleus or adjacent reticular formation, but it is also possible that the section removes a tonic facilitatory influence on more rostral neurones concerned in the reflex arc, as we suggested above for the digastric reflex.

CONCLUSIONS

The relationship between pain and jaw-closing muscle function is therefore not simple, since there seems to be no direct link between high-intensity noxious stimulation and facilitation or excitation of jaw-closing muscles. In fact, the reverse seems to be the case, although we have no information on the responses of the lateral pterygoid, which on clinical evidence is frequently involved in the TMJ pain-dysfunction syndrome. We can, however, speculate on the possible neural mechanisms that underlie masticatory pain conditions such as this syndrome. We know that noxious stimuli can bring about a jaw-opening reflex, and we might argue that the stretching of the jaw-closing muscles thus produced may result in reflex contractions with muscle spasm and pain as possible sequelae. And although these high-intensity stimuli may primarily bring about inhibition of jaw-closing muscles simultaneous with digastric activation, descending higher influences might modify or overcome the inhibitory effects (e.g. Yemm, 1971; Yu et al., 1973).

Pain originating in an arthritic TMJ or in a carious or traumatized tooth may be referred to a muscle by an unknown (possibly cortical) mechanism, which might at the same time disinhibit jaw-closing motoneurones. Thus facilitatory and excitatory influences which are usually masked may become apparent, and so bring about sustained contraction of the muscle and pain.

Alternatively we need not implicate high-threshold afferents at all. Perhaps very small changes in the pattern of excitation of low-threshold afferents from muscles, TMJ, oral mucosa, tongue, and periodontium are sufficient, when summated, to produce excitatory post-synaptic potentials in jaw-closing alpha and gamma motoneurones. The size of these potentials may be increased by the addition of central effects (cortex, cerebellum, reticular formation, etc.). If frank action potentials are produced, the resulting sustained contraction in the muscles could then lead to pain. And, of course, it is not impossible that the phenomenon is entirely centrally induced. But until we have a much more thorough knowledge of the control and regulation of trigeminal motoneurones, or a good experimental animal model for pain-dysfunction syndromes of the oral-facial musculature, we can only speculate.

This work was supported by the Canadian Medical Research Council.

REFERENCES

Achari, N.K., and Thexton, A.J. 1974. A masseteric reflex elicited from the oral mucosa in man. *Archs oral Biol.* 19: 299–302

Anderson, D.J., Hannam, A.G., and Matthews, B. 1970. Sensory mechanisms in mammalian teeth and their supporting structures. *Physiol. Rev.* 50: 171–95

Chase, M.H., Torii, S., and Nakamura, Y. 1970. The influence of vagal afferent fibre activity on masticatory reflexes. *Exp. Neurol.* 27: 545–53

Funakoshi, M., and Amano, N. 1974. Periodontal jaw muscle reflexes in the albino rat. *J. dent. Res.* 53: 598–605

Greenwood, L.F. 1973. An electrophysiological study of the central connections of primary afferent nerve fibres from the dental pulp in the cat. *Archs oral Biol.* 18: 771–85

Greenwood, L.F., and Sessle, B.J. 1973. Identification and peripheral regulation of single trigeminal alpha and gamma motoneurones in the cat. *Proc. 3rd Annual Meeting, Soc. Neurosci.* 45: 10

Hannam, A.G., Siu, W., and Tom, J. 1974. A comparison of monopolar and bipolar pulp testing. *J. Canad. dent. Assoc.* 2: 124–8

Keller, O., Vyklicky, L., and Sykova, E. 1972. Reflexes from Aα and Aδ trigeminal afferents. *Brain Res.* 37: 330–2

Kerr, F. 1972. Central relationships of trigeminal and cervical primary afferents in the spinal cord and medulla. *Brain Res.* 43: 561–72

Kidokoro, Y., Kubota, K., Shuto, S., and Sumino, R. 1968. Reflex organization of cat masticatory muscles. *J. Neurophysiol.* 31: 695–708

Kubota, K., Kidokoro, Y., and Suzuki, J. 1968. Postsynaptic inhibitions of trigeminal and lumbar motoneurones from the superficial radial nerve in the cat. *Jap. J. Physiol.* 18: 198–215

Mahan, P.E., and Anderson, K.V. 1970. Jaw depression elicited by tooth pulp stimulation. *Exp. Neurol.* 29: 439–48

Mehler, W.R. 1969. Some neurological species differences – *a posteriori*. *Ann. N.Y. Acad. Sci.* 167: 424–68

Mosso, J., and Kruger, L. 1973. Receptor categories represented in spinal trigeminal nucleus caudalis. *J. Neurophysiol.* 36: 472–88

Mumford, J. 1965. Pain perception threshold and adaptation of normal human teeth. *Archs oral Biol.* 10: 957–68

Munro, R.R. 1972. Co-ordination of activity of the two bellies of the digastric muscle in basic jaw movements. *J. dent. Res.* 51: 1663–7

Nakamura, Y., Mori, S., and Nagashima, H. 1973. Origin and central pathways of crossed inhibitory effects of afferents from the masseteric muscle on the masseteric motoneurones of the cat. *Brain Res.* 57: 29–42

Nakamura, Y., Wu, C.Y., Nagashima, H., and Mori, S. 1971. Bilaterally symmetrical effects of high threshold afferents from the masseteric muscle on the jaw movement. *Brain Res.* 26: 200–3

Reid, K.H. 1972. Reflex and behavioral withdrawal responses to tooth pulp stimulation. *Proc. 2nd Annual Meeting, Soc. Neurosci.* 15: 6

Riblet, L.A., and Mitchell, C.L. 1972. The effect of cervical spinal section on the ability of morphine to elevate the jaw jerk threshold to electrical stimulation of the tooth pulp in cats. *J. Pharm. Exp. Therap.* 180: 610–15

Schmitt, A., Yu, S.-K.J., and Sessle, B.J. 1973. Excitatory and inhibitory influences from laryngeal and orofacial areas on tongue position in the cat. *Archs oral Biol.* 18: 1121–30

Sessle, B.J., and Greenwood, L.F. 1975. Effects of trigeminal tractotomy and of carbamazepine on single trigeminal sensory neurones in cats. *J. dent. Res.* 54 (Special Issue B): 201B–6B

Sessle, B.J., and Kenny, D.J. 1973. Control of tongue and facial motility: neural mechanisms that may contribute to swallowing and sucking. In J. Bosma (ed.), *Fourth Symposium on Oral Sensation and Perception*. Bethesda: D.H.E.W.

Sherrington, C.S. 1917. Reflexes elicitable in the cat from pinna vibrissae and jaws. *J. Physiol. (Lond.)* 51: 404–31

Sumino, R. 1971. Central neural pathways involved in the jaw-opening reflex in the cat. In R. Dubner and Y. Kawamura (eds.), *Oral-Facial Sensory and Motor Mechanisms*. New York: Appleton-Century-Crofts

Thexton, A.J. 1973. Oral reflexes elicited by mechanical stimulation of palatal mucosa in the cat. *Archs oral Biol.* 18: 971–80

Yemm, R. 1971. A comparison of the electrical activity of masseter and temporal muscles of human subjects during experimental stress. *Archs oral Biol.* 16: 269–73

— 1972. Reflex jaw-opening following electrical stimulation of oral mucous membrane in man. *Archs oral Biol.* 17: 513–23

Yu, S.-K.J., Schmitt, A., and Sessle, B.J. 1973. Inhibitory effects on jaw muscle activity of innocuous and noxious stimulation of facial and intra-oral sites in man. *Archs oral Biol.* 18: 861–70

DISCUSSION

KUBOTA Does pain influence the reflex activity from the so-called flexor reflex afferents? I am not sure whether we know this.

GOLDBERG The jaw-opening reflex can be elicited by stimulation of large-diameter afferent fibres over a wide area of oral mucosa, without the stimulation of the small afferents, even those that exist in the pulp itself.

DUBNER With regard to flexor afferents, I think it is true that some of the flexor reflex afferents are activated by low-threshold stimuli.

MATTHEWS We found that it is impossible to evoke a digastric response in man by electrical stimulation of pulp or mucous membrane. Perhaps this is because with human subjects we are not able to apply sufficiently intense stimuli. In the decerebrate cat one obtains a digastric response at higher stimulus strength than that required for inhibition of elevator activity.

HANNAM We know that the jaw opens actively in a reflex fashion when a hard object is unexpectedly met within a food bolus. Presumably the same sort of thing would happen with a really intense artificial stimulus.

MATTHEWS Yes. It is, of course, easy to produce masseteric inhibition in man with intraoral stimulation, but we have no evidence that it is accompanied by digastric contraction (e.g. Yemm, 1972). While I am on this point, has anyone stimulated tooth pulp electrically in man and looked at the threshold for masseter inhibition and related this to the threshold for sensation? Can you obtain, for example, masseter inhibition at a stimulus intensity below that which produces sensation?

GREENWOOD To my knowledge, no one has studied this, but the problem is that it is only recently that people have even started to differentiate between the first and second period of inhibition. The early inhibition can be produced when there is no unpleasant sensation at all from the intraoral and extraoral tactile receptors (Yu et al., 1973).

THOMAS I may be digressing a bit, but if one takes a transverse section of the motor nerve supplying rat masseter muscle, three kinds of fibres (very large, intermediate, and very small) are found. In the trigeminal motor nucleus there are very small neurones tending to form nests at the ventral end, along with some very much larger ones, which fit the characteristics of alpha and gamma motoneurones. When you cut the motor nerve, you find chromatolysis occurring in both large and small neurones. If you stimulate the motor nucleus directly and record from the masseteric nerve you obtain very slowly conducting, as well as more intermediate and rapidly conducting, potentials. This also indicates the presence of alpha and gamma motoneurones in the motor nucleus.

SESSLE In our extracellular recordings from cells in the trigeminal motor nucleus, Dr Greenwood and I have identified two types of motoneurones. We classify the second as gamma motoneurones on the basis of their higher threshold to antidromic activation, slower conduction velocity, lack of a monosynaptic input on stimulating the trigeminal mesencephalic nucleus, and tonic activity even when the jaw is closed. Jaw-closing alpha motoneurones have a monosynaptic input and never seem to be active in the latter condition. All these characteristics are compatible with those that have been described for spinal gamma motoneurones (e.g. J.C. Eccles et al., *Acta. physiol. scand.* 50 [1960]: 32-40). All in all, I think we do now have definitive evidence that there are gamma motoneurones, at least in the trigeminal motor nucleus. Whether they exist in the other cranial nerve motor nuclei is uncertain. Probably they do not in many, in view of the lack of muscle spindles in most cranial muscles.

GREENWOOD The conduction velocities for both alpha and gamma motoneurones are also quite low. This supports Dr Thomas's observations for trigeminal motoneurones, findings for hypoglossal motoneurones (T. Sumi, *Jap. J. Physiol.* 19 [1969]: 55-67) and facial motoneurones (S.T. Kitai et al., *Brain Res.* 33 [1971]: 227-32). This may be a reflection of the fact that it is difficult to measure the lengths of the conduction paths in those cranial nerves.

MATTHEWS What are they, roughly?

GREENWOOD About 36 mm for the masseter.

MATTHEWS It is a pity the distance is so short.

SESSLE But trigeminal cutaneous afferents may also be slower conducting than their spinal counterparts (e.g. P.R. Burgess et al., *J. Neurophysiol.* 31 [1968]: 833-48; M.J. Rowe and B.J. Sessle, *Brain Res.* 42 [1972]: 367-84).

DUBNER   This may be the case.

DELLOW   To change direction slightly, are there any synapses on the primary sensory neurones in the trigeminal mesencephalic nucleus?

GOBEL   Yes, there are. There are synapses on the cell bodies, but their source is still unknown. At present we suspect they are derived from neurones close by, but they could be from anywhere in the brain stem. One of the problems is that it is very hard to identify small endings with small synaptic vesicles, and this is because they are probably derived from intrinsic neurones, and a nice, clean selective lesion cannot be produced.

SESSLE   This is obviously an area where study is required. It would be relatively simple to record from the mesencephalic nucleus and have electrodes in a number of various nerves and areas of the brain to see if the discharge of the mesencephalic neurones could be affected. That would give one some idea of whether there is a modulating influence. But, of course, the synapses may serve a neurotrophic or metabolic influence. For example, it has been shown that the number of synapses varies with the age of the animal (e.g. K.E. Alley, *J. Embryol. exp. Morph.* 31 [1974] : 99–121).

GOBEL   I should also add that we know that the primary afferent endings on ventral horn motoneurones have axoaxonic synapses, and this may well turn out to be the case for primary afferents to the cranial motor nuclei.

Chairman's Summary

R. DUBNER

Pain in the oral-facial region may originate from many different sources: tooth, oral mucosa, gingiva or periodontal membrane, bone or joint, muscle, etc. Acute pain arising from these multiple sources is usually accompanied by a protective jaw-opening reflex involving excitation of jaw-opening muscles and inhibition of jaw-closing muscles. It also is known that a jaw-opening reflex can be evoked by non-noxious stimuli such as tooth tap or tactile stimuli applied to the oral mucosa. Therefore, jaw opening or simple digastric muscle activity cannot be considered a signal of the presence of noxious input. Reid (1972) also has shown that escape levels in the cat occur at 2 to 5 times the threshold required to produce jaw opening evoked by tooth pulp stimulation.

Are there any distinct characteristics of the protective jaw-opening reflex produced by noxious stimuli when compared to the jaw-opening reflex evoked by innocuous stimuli? The evidence presented in this section indicates that there are a number of differences. Noxious stimulation of the human lip produces complete or partial inhibition of masseter muscle activity which has a more variable and longer duration than that produced by innocuous stimuli and includes a late inhibitory period (Yu, Schmitt, and Sessle, 1973). This late inhibitory period appears to involve a reflex pathway which relays in trigeminal nucleus caudalis (Riblet and Mitchell, 1972) or in trigeminal nucleus interpolaris and adjacent reticular formation (Sumino, 1971). On the other hand, innocuous natural and mild electrical stimuli appear to produce inhibition of jaw-closing muscles via a pathway involving the supratrigeminal nucleus in the pons (Kidokoro et al., 1968; Sumino, 1971; Yu et al., 1973). These early and late inhibitory periods may involve different synaptic mechanisms. The early inhibition clearly results from postsynaptic inhibitory mechanisms, whereas the late inhibitory period has some characteristics of presynaptic inhibition (Sumino, 1971).

A final difference between the protective jaw-opening reflex and that evoked by innocuous stimuli is the central control pathways influencing each reflex. Recent evidence indicates that the jaw-opening reflex elicited by tooth pulp stimulation is inhibited from different midbrain sites than the reflex evoked by tooth tap (Oliveras et al., 1974). It is also of interest that inhibition of jaw-closing muscles can be overridden by high levels of maintained voluntary muscle activity (Yu et al., 1973). In cases of temporomandibular joint pain-dysfunction there is often increased activity and spasm of jaw-closing muscles which apparently has 'swamped' the protective inhibitory reflex evoked by activation of nociceptive muscle afferents (Matthews, 1972).

At this point one might ask the question: what can we learn from studying the parameters of the jaw-opening reflex that would help to improve our understanding of pathological pain? I believe that we can improve our diagnostic procedures and better determine aetiological factors and foci by studying simple reflex activity during function. At what stages of chewing and swallowing are different reflexes maximized? Thexton (1974) has shown that jaw position influences the type of reflex evoked by a particular intensity of electrical stimulation. A preliminary step to increasing our understanding of the role of simpler reflexes during function is the study of such reflexes in isolation. I believe we have reached the stage where an analysis of such reflexes during complex masticatory functions in awake, behaving animals, and in humans, can be pursued.

REFERENCES

Kidokoro, Y., Kubota, K., Shuto, S., and Sumino, R. 1968. Reflex organization of masticatory muscles in the cat. *J. Neurophysiol.* 31: 695–708
Matthews, P.B.C. 1972. *Mammalian Muscle Receptors and their Central Actions*. Baltimore: Williams and Wilkins
Oliveras, J.L., Woda, A., Guilbaud, G., and Besson, J.M. 1974. Inhibition of the jaw-opening reflex by electrical stimulation of the periaqueductal grey matter in the awake, unrestrained cat. *Brain Res.* 72: 328–31
Reid, K.H. 1972. Reflex and behavioral withdrawal responses to tooth pulp stimulation. *Proc. 2nd Annual Meeting, Soc. Neurosci.* 15: 6
Riblet, L.A., and Mitchell, C.L. 1972. The effect of cervical spinal section on the ability of morphine to elevate the jaw jerk threshold to electrical stimulation of the tooth pulp in cats. *J. Pharmacol. exp. Therap.* 180: 610–15
Sumino, R. 1971. Central neural pathways involved in the jaw-opening reflex in the cat. In R. Dubner and Y. Kawamura (eds.), *Oral-Facial Sensory and Motor Mechanisms*. New York: Appleton-Century-Crofts
Thexton, A.J. 1974. Jaw opening and jaw closing reflexes in the cat. *Brain Res.* 66: 425–33
Yu, S.-K.J., Schmitt, A., and Sessle, B.J. 1973. Inhibitory effects on jaw muscle activity of innocuous and noxious stimulation of facial and intraoral sites in man. *Archs oral Biol.* 18: 861–70

SECTION FOUR

Mastication and swallowing:
Patterning and controls of muscle activity

Chairman's Introduction

A.G. HANNAM

We shall approach mastication and swallowing from a more behavioural point of view in this section. In human studies, we are only permitted to observe the systems in normal function, or to perturb them in a limited fashion in order to measure the effect of the perturbation on the few parameters we are able to quantitate. We can measure, for example, the modalities and intensities of sensation reported by the subject, and the manifestations of motoneurone activity, in the form of electromyographic signals, generated forces, or displacement. Even so, there are a surprising number of experimental approaches available to us. Many of these are in themselves not technically demanding, yet given the vast number of questions which need answering from the behavioural aspect, it is sad that we have such a small amount of information available at present.

Much of the original work done in the psychophysical field has concentrated upon measuring such perceptual skills as the ability of subjects to detect the thickness of objects held between the teeth (Kawamura and Watanabe, 1960), the forces applied to the teeth (Bowman and Nakfoor, 1968), and the shapes of objects held in the mouth (Shelton, Arndt, and Hetherington, 1967). The assessment of motor performance has generally been limited to studies involving the measurement of bite force under different conditions (Carlsson, 1974) where most of the emphasis has been placed upon the forces produced, rather than upon the methods used by the organism to produce them. In the masticatory system, closed-loop studies of the sort frequently found in the literature on swallowing, where both input and output are observed and perhaps manipulated in the intact organism, are relatively rare. In this regard the work of Wennström (1971, 1972) is notable. His experiments on the ability of the human subject to grade voluntarily bite force under different constraints have shown us, for example, that at low bite levels, we are capable of discriminating light bite force changes, but that with stronger bites, greater force changes are required to obtain equal discrimination. In similar experiments in our laboratory, we have recently been able to demonstrate that the presence of a periodic anchor or reference force, even if this is simply referred to as 'maximum comfortable bite,' significantly improves a subject's grading performance over that exhibited when he relates on a longer term, more abstract, reference. Later in this section, Dr Lund will discuss the role of peripheral feedback in the generation of graded bite force, and in doing so introduces us to a more sophisticated type of closed-loop experiment, involving the use of tracking tasks and perturbations. It is this sort of approach that holds a great deal of promise in studies of the human masticatory system, both in the examination of reflex behaviour and in the observation of adaptive, learning phenomena.

With the exception of elegant cinefluorographic techniques of the kind used by Cleall (1965), electromyography and the measurement of jaw displacement have been the most widely used methods of studying chewing and swallowing in man under normal, or near-normal, conditions. The well-known basic electromyographic studies of Ahlgren (1966) and Møller (1966) hardly need mentioning, and we are fortunate to have Dr Møller's contribution to this symposium. We have derived a lot of information about muscle function from this work, and we are now beginning to witness a trend towards applying the basic methodology, so carefully established by Møller, to cases involving skeletal abnormalities, suspected abnormalities of muscle function, and dental malocclusion. At the same time, technology has permitted advances to be made in the study of jaw movement in normal function. Since Ahlgren's efforts to record jaw movement in more than one plane (Ahlgren, 1966), more studies have begun to appear in which serious efforts have been made to quantitate displacement patterns in three dimensions (Gibbs et al., 1971; Gillings, Graham, and Duckmanton, 1973; Griffin and Malor, 1974) and we now have to deal with new parameters such as angles of the approach and departure pathways, velocity, and acceleration.

Despite a good, and increasing amount of electromyographic data, and despite a promising increase in our knowledge of displacement patterns, there is at present a marked lack of data which directly relates muscle function to jaw displacement under normal conditions of behaviour. A limited study by Ahlgren (1967) is about all we have at the moment. Sophisticated displacement transducers, and multichannel electromyographic recording do, of course, create their own data acquisition and handling problems, not to mention the problems of devising statistical methods suitable for extracting some meaning from the data. In conclusion, one might cautiously predict that, during the next few years, digital sampling techniques and the use of computer technology will provide much of the data we need. How we devise our experiments, and how we interpret the results in terms of the behaviour of the neuromuscular system in chewing and swallowing is another problem altogether.

REFERENCES

Ahlgren, J. 1966. Mechanism of mastication. *Acta odont. scand.* 24: suppl. 44
– 1967. Pattern of chewing and malocclusion of the teeth. *Acta odont. scand.* 25: 3-13
Bowman, D.C., and Nakfoor, P.M. 1968. Evaluation of the human subject's ability to differentiate intensity of forces applied to the maxillary central incisors. *J. dent. Res.* 47: 252-9
Carlsson, G.E. 1974. Bite force and chewing efficiency. In Y. Kawamura (ed.), *Frontiers of Oral Physiology.* Vol. 1. *Physiology of Mastication.* Basel: Karger
Cleall, J.F. 1965. Deglutition. A study of form and function. *Am. J. Orthodont.* 51: 566-94
Gibbs, C.H., Messerman, T., Reswick, J.B., and Derda, H.J. 1971. Functional movements of the mandible. *J. prosth. Dent.* 26: 604-20
Gillings, B.R.D., Graham, C.H., and Duckmanton, N.A. 1973. Jaw movements in young adult men during chewing. *J. prosth. Dent.* 29: 616-27
Griffin, C.J., and Malor, R. 1974. An analysis of mandibular movements. In Y. Kawamura (ed.), *Frontiers of Oral Physiology.* Vol. 1. *Physiology of Mastication.* Basel: Karger
Kawamura, Y., and Watanabe, M. 1960. Studies of oral sensory thresholds: the discrimination of small differences in thickness of steel wires in persons with natural and artificial dentitions. *Med. J. Osaka Univ.* 10: 291-301
Møller, E. 1966. The chewing apparatus. *Acta physiol. scand.* 69: suppl. 280
Shelton, R.L., Arndt, W.B., and Hetherington, J.J. 1967. Testing oral stereognosis. In J.F. Bosma (ed.), *Symposium on Oral Sensation and Perception.* Springfield, Ill.: Thomas
Wennström, A. 1971. Psychophysical investigation of bite force. Part I. *Sven. Tandläk T.* 64: 807-19
– 1972. Psychophysical investigation of bite force. Part III. *Sven. Tandläk T.* 65: 177-84

Human muscle patterns

EIGILD MØLLER

Mastication and swallowing are examples of motor performances subject to analysis in man and animal at different steps. Muscle activity represents an intermediary phase linking nervous processing which is based on inherent activity, stored information, and acute sensations, with force and movement, and comminution and transfer of food. Electromyography can disclose motor patterns at various levels: coordination of groups of muscles, activity in individual muscles as a whole or as discrete parts, and even in motor units. This report aims to specify traits in the coordination of the muscles of mastication of common significance to neurophysiology and clinical dentistry.

MASTICATION

During natural mastication the main part of a bolus is kept together and shifted at random from right to left within the same sequence of strokes or from one sequence to the next (Møller, 1966, 1974; Wictorin, Hedegård, and Lundberg, 1968). Therefore, the pattern of muscle activity averaged from a number of strokes during natural chewing will normally be an artefact. A true pattern can be obtained during deliberate unilateral chewing on the right or left side; specification of muscle activity in relation to placement of bolus is required.

Bilateral patterns of mandibular elevators

The coordination of the elevators (Møller, 1966, 1974) is strongly influenced by the position of the bolus, and according to the response in this respect they fall into two groups: (1) the anterior and posterior temporal muscles characterized by an earlier activation on the side of the bolus (ipsilateral) as compared with the contralateral side. Bolus placement is reflected slightly in the intensity of the activity in the anterior part of the muscle (strongest ipsilaterally), but normally not in the more horizontal posterior fibres; (2) the masseter and medial pterygoid muscles in which the activity is related to bolus placement by its intensity with strong ipsilateral predominance. Their timing shows more or less pronounced differences in the opposite direction to the temporal, with the contralateral muscles leading.

Timing of the elevators reveals basic features of mandibular movements. Vertical movements are associated with almost synchronous activation, while large transverse excursions imply an enlarged time dispersal between leading and retarded muscles (Møller, 1974, Fig. 18).

Quantitative evaluation of the pattern of bilateral activity in the elevators (Møller, 1974, Figs. 9 and 10) can be applied clinically to decide whether or not chewing is performed with the normal shift of bolus. Consistent restriction to the same side signifies functional asymmetry of muscle activity and mandibular movements that may become permanent. The patterns denote appropriate directions of movements to be improved and may contribute to control of treatment (Møller, 1969, Fig. 5).

Activity in the elevators during individual chewing strokes

Transient inhibition
Mechanical stimulation of single teeth, tapping the teeth together, and mastication may result in transient inhibition of the elevators visible in electromyographic recordings (Fig. 1). Evidence on the origin and pathways for this inhibition is conflicting. Sessle and Schmitt (1972) claim to have proved that activation of periodontal receptors is the sole cause. However, oral tactile sensibility has been shown to be reduced markedly during chewing when compared to that measured during conscious biting (Öwall and Møller, 1974), and similarly the reflex responses to artificial stimulation of the teeth may not be the same as those occurring during mastication. Furthermore, the inhibitory periods noted by Sessle and Schmitt (1972), as well as those observed by Goldberg (1971), were preceded by facilitation. Application of a mechanical stimulus to the palatal mucosa also results in facilitation (Thexton, 1973). Therefore, the actual response to natural stimulation of periodontal and mucosal mechanoreceptors may be a facilitation comparable to the supporting reaction elicited by touching the skin of the foot (magnet reaction [Roberts, 1967]). It fits with this assumption that the elevators act most strongly close to or in the intercuspal position (Møller, 1966), a position characterized by maximal support for the generation of force.

Transient inhibitory periods in the elevators during mastication (Ahlgren, 1969; Hannam, Matthews, and Yemm, 1969) have been demonstrated by Öwall and Elmquist (1974) during two conditions: when closing movements

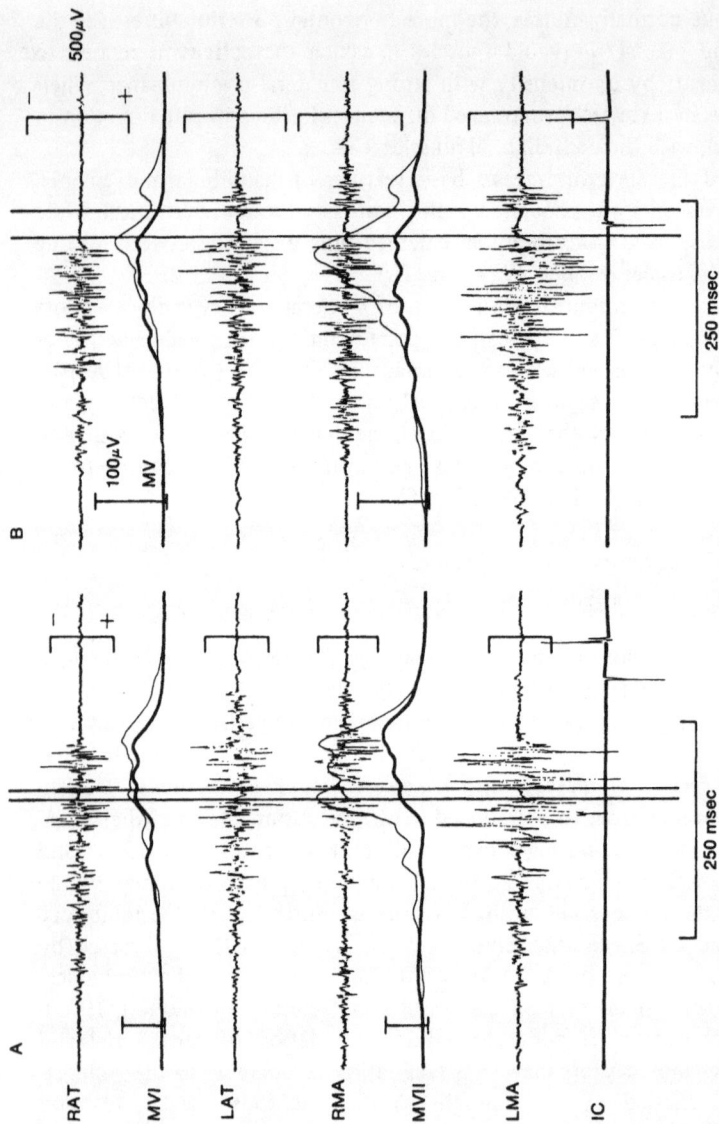

FIGURE 1   Transient inhibitions in a left-sided stroke recorded during natural chewing of peanuts (A) and deliberate left-sided chewing of gum (B). Records show electrical activity in the right and left anterior temporal (RAT, LAT) and masseter muscles (RMA, LMA), the corresponding mean voltages (MV I and II, heavy trace: right muscle, thin trace: left muscle), and incisor contact (IC; downwards deflection: make, upwards deflection: break). Vertical lines delineate periods of transient inhibition. Note: during natural chewing, transient inhibition precedes incisor contact by 250 msec; during unilateral chewing of gum, inhibition and make of contact coincide. Surface electrodes; male 24 years old; copy in indian ink from ultraviolet recording (courtesy of B. Öwall and E. Møller).

were abruptly arrested, or abruptly released. In relation to occlusion, inhibition due to sudden stops and to unloading become features with clinical relevance, and are reflected in the pattern of the elevator muscles. The reflex response to afferent activity from muscle spindles and tendon organs (Matthews, 1972), and the simultaneous activation of alpha and gamma motoneurones demonstrated by activity in spindle afferents during active contraction (Taylor and Davey, 1968; Vallbo, 1970), may account for the inhibitory mechanism.

Inhibition due to stop of jaw movement
If shortening of an elevator is delayed or arrested, gamma efferent activity will impose stretch upon the nuclear bag region of the intrafusal fibres. The result is increased facilitation of the alpha motoneurones, resulting in stronger contraction to overcome resistance. If the stop is definitive, rapidly increasing tension of the isometric contraction will activate tendon organs and cause inhibition. Tendon organs have extremely low thresholds to active contraction and are connected to fractions of different motor units. Thus the input from the population of tendon organs in a muscle is a measure of the total forces produced; in addition, the tendon organ has a distinct dynamic component and will react more than proportionally to rapid increases in tension (Houk and Henneman, 1967). Such a situation exists during mastication when the mandible is stopped, and it is exaggerated by the initial facilitation of alpha motor fibres to overcome resistance. The reaction could be due to a hard particle in the food or interference of a cusp not permitting displacement of the mandible.

Inhibition due to unloading
During biting, unloading may occur if a bolus suddenly gives way (Hannam, Matthews, and Yemm, 1968; Öwall and Elmquist, 1974). If a muscle shortens too fast, the spindles are unloaded, their facilitating afferent activity is abolished, and inhibition (disfacilitation) results. Angel and colleagues (1965, 1973) have suggested this mechanism. They demonstrated that a certain amount of shortening was required to obtain inhibition, and excluded discharges from tendon organs and Renshaw cells or stretch of the antagonist as alternative sources of inhibition. During chewing, unloading of the elevators may be due to a brittle bolus or cusp interferences permitting displacement.

Terminal inhibition and transfer to opening
If activity from periodontal receptors was responsible for terminal inhibition of the anterior temporal muscle, a correlation could be expected between the time course or the intensity of its activity and the 'make' of tooth contact.

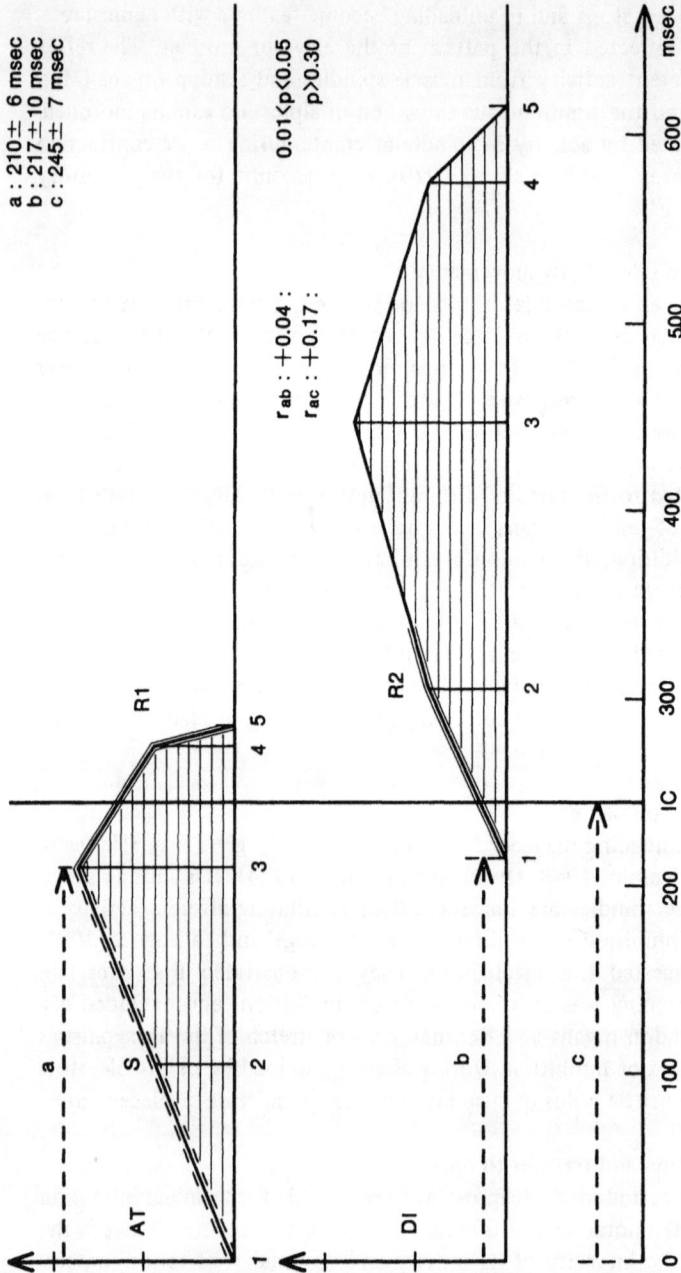

FIGURE 2 Mechanism of transfer from closing to opening in a chewing stroke. Diagrammatic presentation of average time course of the activity in the anterior temporal (AT) and digastric muscles (DI) and the make of incisor contact (IC, vertical line) during a single chewing stroke. a: time to maximal activity in AT; b: time to onset of activity in DI; c: time to onset of activity in AT; time to IC. r_{ab} and r_{ac}: coefficients of correlation (product-moment). 1: onset of activity; 2–4: time to 50%, 100%, and decline to 50% maximum mean voltage; 5: cessation of activity. Time zero: onset of activity in AT. S: adequate stimulus of tendon organs in AT. R1 and R2: response to afferent activity from tendon organs. Note positive correlation between a and b and absence of correlation between a and c. Data from Møller, 1966.

Such a correlation does not exist (Møller, 1966, Table 18). Instead, the time of maximal activity in the anterior temporal muscle coincides with the onset of activity in the digastric muscle (Fig. 2). Biological interpretation of this coincidence is possible by considering the reflex effect of activating the tendon organs of the elevator muscles. The increase of activity in the anterior temporal muscle during mastication represents the adequate stimulus of its tendon organs, while the subsequent decrease of activity in this muscle and the increase of activity in the digastric muscle indicate the reflex response. The delay between mechanical and electrical activity implies that the tension necessary to produce inhibition must be below peak tension in the chewing stroke.

The previous discussion assumes normal supporting tissues and even distribution of the forces of mastication. Inflammation and deficient occlusion may result in periodontal pressure surpassing pain threshold and causing inhibition by a different mechanism.

Recruitment of motor units

In mammalian muscle three types of muscle fibres are distinguished: *type A*, which have a high content of myofibrillar ATPase and low content of mitochondrial ATPase, contract fast and are easily fatigued; *type C*, with reversed content of myofibrillar and mitochondrial ATPase and which contract slowly and are resistant to fatigue; and *type B*, with intermediary histochemical and mechanical properties. Within a motor unit all fibres are of uniform type (Henneman and Olsson, 1965; Edström and Kugelberg, 1968; Burke et al., 1971). Twitch tension of motor units with type A fibres is 4-5 times larger than that of type C motor units (Edström and Kugelberg, 1968). Tetanic tension of type A units exceeds that of type C units by a factor of 12 (Burke et al., 1971). In human muscles with fibres predominantly type A or C, average contraction times differ from the properties of these fibres in animals (Buchthal and Schmalbruch, 1970).

Fibres histochemically typed as A are suited for strong, phasic activity (e.g. mastication) and type C for sustained postural activity. That altered functional demands may result in changes of histochemical composition and size of skeletal muscle fibres (Guth and Yellin, 1971) led Ringquist (1974) to compare biopsy specimens from the temporal muscle of dentate subjects and denture wearers. Specimens from the internal surface had fewer type A fibres in denture wearers as compared with fully dentate subjects. A similar difference was true for both the internal and external surfaces when dentate subjects were compared with patients with clinically deficient dentures; in addition, dissatisfied denture wearers had smaller type A fibres than subjects who considered their dentures adequate. (Fibres denoted type 1 and 2 by Ringquist are equivalent respectively to type C and A mentioned above.)

In dentate subjects as well as in contented and dissatisfied denture wearers, fibres histochemically typed as C had the same size (Ringquist, 1974). Since the temporal muscle supports the mandible at rest (Lous, Sheik-Ol-Eslam, and Møller, 1970; Møller, Sheik-Ol-Eslam, and Lous, 1971), this observation is in keeping with a similar demand for sustained, postural activity irrespective of dentitional state. It indicates recruitment of different motor units in posture and mastication.

'Phase-angles' in the chewing cycle

Patterns of activity in the muscles moving the mandible divides the chewing stroke into three phases (Fig. 3): (1) opening, with predominance alternating between the ipsilateral and contralateral digastric muscles; (2) closing, with predominance first of the ipsilateral, then of the contralateral posterior temporal muscle; and (3) a phase displaced 90° in relation to the previous position with the ipsilateral, lateral pterygoid acting strongest in the last half of closing and the first half of opening and the contralateral, lateral pterygoid dominating from half-open to half-closed.

This intricate pattern is related to incisor occlusion: subjects with marked overbite have strong activity in the posterior temporal muscles and an exaggerated overlap in time between these muscles and the lateral pterygoid and digastric muscles (Møller, 1974, Figs 19 and 24). Both features are interpreted as means to obtain precise guiding of the mandible.

Patterns of activity in the lips

Surface electromyograms from the lips are compound recordings from different, separately innervated muscles (Møller, 1966; Blanton, Briggs, and Perkins, 1970). Strongest activity occurs during the opening movement (primary activity) to produce an anterior seal (orbicularis oris) and to position the bolus between the teeth (buccinator), but the lips are also active during closing (secondary activity). Recordings made with wire electrodes from individual muscles (Fig. 4) show that the secondary activity in the upper lip originates from its levator muscle for the purpose of withdrawal.

The degree of primary activity in the lower lip during mastication is related to facial prognathism. In subjects with retrognathism of both jaws the lips are usually sufficient and the anterior seal demands slight activity; with prognathism the lower lip may be taut at rest and chewing requires strong activity

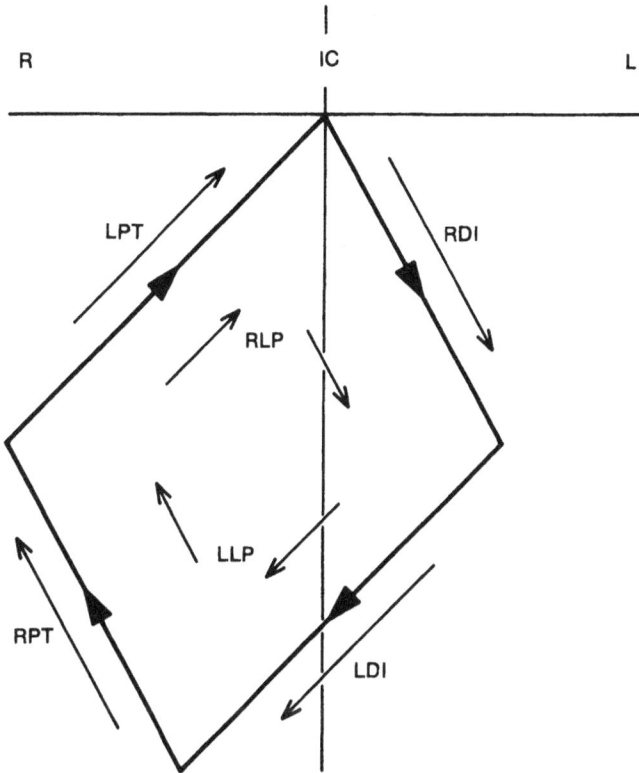

FIGURE 3 Phases of movement and muscle activity in a right-sided chewing stroke. R: right side, L: left side, IC: intercuspal position. The trapezium represents movements of the lower incisors in a frontal plane seen facing the subject; superimposed arrows indicate direction of movement. Separate arrows signify predominance of the different muscles moving the mandible: right and left digastric (RDI, LDI), right and left posterior temporal (RPT, LPT) and right and left lateral pterygoid muscles (RLP, LLP). Note that RLP/LLP are activated with a phase angle of 90° relative to RDI/LDI and RPT/LPT. Diagram based on average data from Møller, 1966.

(Møller, 1966, Fig. 81). The relation between lip function and facial morphology exemplifies an important feature: the lips adjust the oral cavity to the particular function being performed (mastication, swallowing, speech) and are primarily activated to produce their own movements. The adaptive function seems to depend more on recognition of the shape of the supporting hard tissues than on the tension produced. The exteroceptive reflex control of facial muscles (Lindquist, 1973) is in keeping with this assumption.

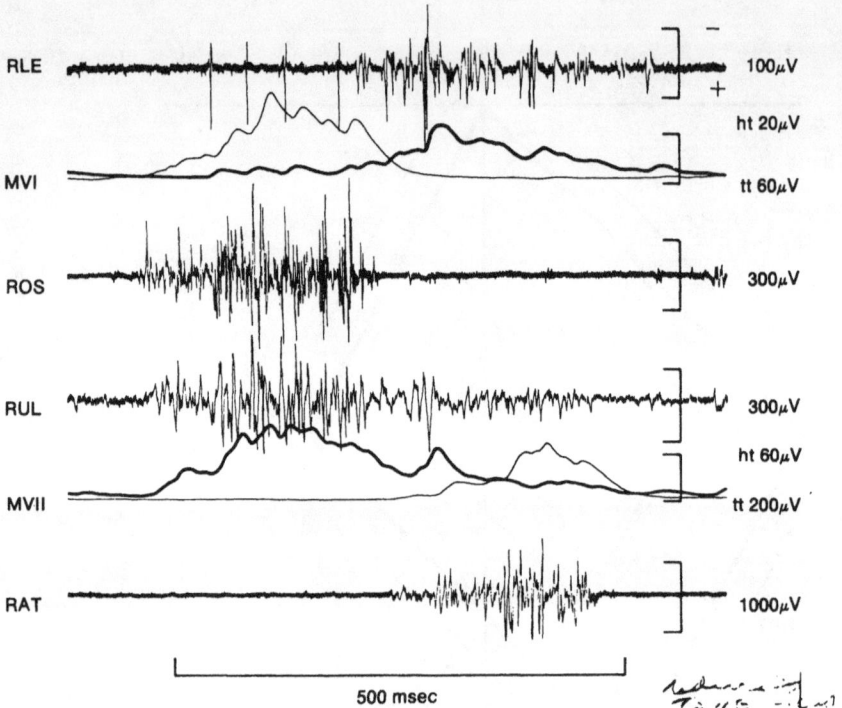

FIGURE 4 Discrete and compound recordings from the upper lip during deliberate left-sided mastication. Electrical activity in the right upper levator and orbicularis oris (RLE/ROS), in the right upper lip as a whole (RUL) and in the right anterior temporal muscle (RAT). MV I: mean voltage of RLE (heavy trace, ht) and ROS (thin trace, tt); MV II: mean voltage of RUL (heavy trace) and RAT (thin trace). The activity in RAT indicates closing. Note in the compound recording (RUL) that the activity during opening originates from ROS and during closing from RLE. RLE and ROS recorded with bipolar intramuscular wire electrodes, RUL and RAT with bipolar surface electrodes; male 28 years old; copy in indian ink from ultraviolet recording (courtesy of S. Fibiger).

SWALLOWING

Muscle coordination

Swallowing is characterized by synergistic activation of the muscles of mastication with systematic differences between pairs of muscles at the onset of activity (Møller, 1966, Fig. 44 A and B). The elevators start with intervals of about 50 msec; first the medial pterygoid, then the temporal, and finally the

masseter muscle. The lateral pterygoids begin in time with the medial pterygoids, i.e. early in the sequence. Mylohyoid and digastric muscles are activated
simultaneously (in time with the temporal muscle), but the time course of
their activity differs. The mylohyoid muscles contributing to tongue movements in the oral phase by stabilizing the hyoid bone contract strongly from
the onset. In the digastric muscles, activity is moderate for the first 150 msec,
and then strong action moves the hyoid bone and larynx forward and upward.
The genioglossus and geniohyoid muscles have a similar time dispersal of
strong activity (Cunningham and Basmajian, 1969). The muscles of the lips
start early in the oral phase (in time with the pterygoid muscles) to establish
an anterior seal.

Analysis of correlation between the degree of activity in the different muscles during swallowing of saliva (Møller, 1966, Table 23) indicates a division
into three groups: (1) anterior and posterior temporal and masseter muscles,
(2) digastric and mylohyoid muscles, and (3) muscles of the lips. The pterygoid muscles are correlated with both elevators and depressors. The activity in
the three groups varies independently, with no evidence of a specifically large
action of the lips in subjects with low activity in the elevators. However, during swallowing of food a negative correlation between the maximal mean voltage in one of the elevators (anterior temporal) and the upper lip has been demonstrated in children with normal occlusion (Ingervall and Thilander, 1974).

Tooth contact

Over 60 per cent of adults and children swallow with regular tooth contact.
In accordance with the early onset of activity in the lateral pterygoid muscles,
contact is first made with the mandible protruded, followed by a slide into
the intercuspal position.

Subjects swallowing without tooth contact have less activity in their temporal and masseter muscles (25%) than subjects with tooth contact. However,
the degree of activity in the masseter muscle is a poor indicator of tooth contact except in the few subjects with very strong activity (Møller, 1966, Fig.
59). All other muscles display the same degree of activity whether tooth contact occurs or not.

Coordination of tongue and lips

Electromyography
Lip and tongue activity in subjects with a different relationship between the
length of the lips and the anterior height of the alveolar and dental arches
point to a common mechanism of control (Møller, 1966, Fig. 83). With suffi-

cient lip length only slight activity is necessary to establish the anterior seal. Moderate insufficiency is compensated for by increased activity. However, with obvious insufficiency of the lips the pattern changes drastically: the lips remain passive while the tongue, indicated by the activity in the mylohyoid muscle, acts earlier. Reversely, an extremely late onset of activity in the mylohyoid muscle and thus in the tongue requires intense activation of the lips in spite of sufficient lip closure at rest.

Cinefluorography
Protrusion of the tongue to contact the lips may occur during swallowing in subjects with malocclusion and with normal occlusion (Cleall, 1965), and also physiologically (Milne and Cleall, 1970). In subjects with maxillary overjet, anterior seal is often obtained by intrusion of the lower lip between upper and lower incisors and protrusion of the tongue, but after correction of incisor occlusion these features may disappear (Subtelny, 1970, Figs 14 and 15). Attempts aimed primarily at changing swallowing by exercises have no significant effect on tongue behaviour or malocclusion (Subtelny, 1970). However, cinefluorography is a biased approach to the function-form relationship: that lip and tongue morphologically fit with malocclusion and after treatment with normal occlusion does not immediately signify that an exaggerating, abnormal pattern has turned into a stabilizing, harmonious one.

Nervous regulation of function to form

Patterns of interaction between lips and tongue in subjects with various degrees of facial prognathism (Møller, 1966), with transient or permanent open bite (Cleall, 1965; Milne and Cleall, 1970) or maxillary overjet before and after treatment (Subtelny, 1970) exemplify functional adaptation. Because of feedback in terms of tension, this adaptation may compensate for differences in basal morphology by aligning the incisors in normal relationship or it may exaggerate malocclusion.

In the cat, reflex control of the intrinsic muscles of the tongue depends on feedback from receptors in the lingual mucosa (Lindquist and Mårtensson, 1969), i.e. a mechanism similar to that controlling the action of lip and cheek muscles. It is suggested that in man adaptation of lip and tongue function is also exteroceptive and based on activity from mucosal receptors processed in the central nervous system to a neurophysiological image of morphology. Oral function specified in terms of muscle coordination, receptor activity, and central processing can open this image to objective assessment.

REFERENCES

Ahlgren, J. 1969. The silent period in the EMG of the jaw muscles during mastication and its relationship to tooth contact. *Acta odont. scand.* 27: 219-27

Angel, R.W., Eppler, W., and Iannone, A. 1965. Silent period produced by unloading of muscle during voluntary contraction. *J. Physiol. (Lond.)* 180: 864-70

Angel, R.W., Garland, H., and Moore, W. 1973. Unloading reflex during blockade of antagonist muscle nerves. *Electroenceph. clin. Neurophysiol.* 34: 303-7

Blanton, P.L., Briggs, N.L., and Perkins, R.C. 1970. Electromyographic analysis of the buccinator muscle. *J. dent. Res.* 49: 389-94

Buchthal, F., and Schmalbruch, H. 1970. Contraction times and fibre types in intact human muscle. *Acta physiol. scand.* 79: 435-52

Burke, R.E., Levine, D.N., Zajac III, F.E., Tsairis, P., and Engel, W.K. 1971. Mammalian motor units: physiological - histochemical correlation in three types in cat gastrocnemius. *Science* 174: 709-12

Cleall, J.F. 1965. Deglutition: a study of form and function. *Am. J. Orthodont.* 51: 566-94

Cunningham, D.P., and Basmajian, J.V. 1969. Electromyography of genio-glossus and geniohyoid muscles during deglutition. *Anat. Rec.* 165: 401-10

Edström, L., and Kugelberg, E. 1968. Histochemical composition, distribution of fibres and fatiguability of single motor units. Anterior tibial muscle of the rat. *J. Neurol. Neurosurg. Psychiat.* 31: 424-33

Goldberg, L.J. 1971. Masseter muscle excitation induced by stimulation of periodontal and gingival receptors in man. *Brain Res.* 32: 369-81

Guth, L., and Yellin, H. 1971. The dynamic nature of so-called 'fiber types' of mammalian skeletal muscle. *Exp. Neurol.* 31: 277-300

Hannam, A.G., Matthews, B., and Yemm, R. 1968. The unloading reflex in masticatory muscles of man. *Archs oral Biol.* 13: 361-4

- 1969. Changes in the activity of the masseter muscle following tooth contact in man. *Archs oral Biol.* 14: 1401-6

Henneman, E., and Olson, C.B. 1965. Relations between structure and function in the design of skeletal muscles. *J. Neurophysiol.* 28: 581-98

Houk, J., and Henneman, E. 1967. Responses of Golgi tendon organs to active contractions of the soleus muscle of the cat. *J. Neurophysiol.* 30: 466-81

Ingervall, B., and Thilander, B. 1974. Relation between facial morphology and activity of the masticatory muscles. *J. oral Rehab.* 1: 131-47

Lindquist, C. 1973. Reflex organization and contraction properties of facial muscles. An experimental study in the cat. *Acta physiol. scand.* suppl. 393

Lindquist, C., and Mårtensson, A. 1969. Reflex responses induced by stimulation of hypoglossal afferents. *Acta physiol. scand.* 77: 234–40

Lous, I., Sheik-Ol-Eslam, A., and Møller, E. 1970. Postural activity in subjects with functional disorders of the chewing apparatus. *Scand. J. dent. Res.* 78: 404–10

Matthews, P.B.C. 1972. *Mammalian Muscle Receptors and Their Central Actions.* London: Arnold

Milne, I.M., and Cleall, J.F. 1970. Cinefluorographic study of functional adaptation of oro-pharyngeal structures. *Angle Orthodont.* 40: 267–83

Møller, E. 1966. The chewing apparatus. An electromyographic study of the action of the muscles of mastication and its correlation to facial morphology. *Acta physiol. scand.* 69: suppl. 280

– 1969. Clinical electromyography in dentistry. *Int. dent. J.* 19: 250–66

– 1974. Action of the muscles of mastication. In Y. Kawamura (ed.), *Frontiers of Oral Physiology.* Vol. 1. *Physiology of Mastication.* Basel: Karger

Møller, E., Sheik-Ol-Eslam, A., and Lous, I. 1971. Deliberate relaxation of the temporal and masseter muscles in subjects with functional disorders of the chewing apparatus. *Scand. J. dent. Res.* 79: 478–82

Öwall, B., and Elmquist, D. 1974. Motor pauses in EMG activity during chewing and biting. In B. Öwall, *Studies on Oral Perception during Chewing. Odont. Revy* 25: suppl. 28

Öwall, B., and Møller, E. 1974. Oral tactile sensibility during biting and chewing. In B. Öwall, *Studies on Oral Perception during Chewing. Odont. Revy* 25: suppl. 28

Ringquist, M. 1974. A histochemical study of temporal muscle fibers in denture wearers and subjects with natural dentition. *Scand. J. dent. Res.* 82: 28–39

Roberts, T.D.M. 1967. *Neurophysiology of Postural Mechanisms.* London: Butterworths

Sessle, B.J., and Schmitt, A. 1972. Effects of controlled tooth stimulation on jaw muscle activity in man. *Archs oral Biol.* 17: 1597–607

Subtelny, J.D. 1970. Malocclusions, orthodontic corrections and orofacial muscle adaptation. *Angle Orthodont.* 40: 170–201

Taylor, A., and Davey, M.R. 1968. Behaviour of jaw muscle stretch receptors during active and passive movements in the cat. *Nature* 220: 301–2

Thexton, A.J. 1973. Oral reflexes elicited by mechanical stimulation of palatal mucosa in the cat. *Archs oral Biol.* 18: 971–80

Vallbo, Å.B. 1970. Discharge patterns in human spindle afferents during isometric voluntary contractions. *Acta physiol. scand.* 80: 552-66

Wictorin, L., Hedegård, B., and Lundberg, M. 1968. Masticatory function –
A cineradiographic study. III. Position of bolus in individuals with full
complement of natural teeth. *Acta odont. scand.* 26: 213-22

DISCUSSION

ROYDHOUSE   One small point. I notice that Møller states that the lips form
an anterior seal during mastication. Mastication with the lips closed may be
solely a function of the social environment. Small children masticate with
their mouths open, and movies (Univ. of Adelaide) made of Australian abori-
ginals during eating show that these people also eat with their mouths open.

STOREY I think we have to be careful here about racial differences. The
Nubians I have been studying with Harris's research team from Michigan, do
the same. However, what Møller says is right for his group and is probably
also true for the North American population during chewing and swallowing.

LOWE   Since the mylohyoid muscle is not a true extrinsic tongue muscle and
is primarily involved with raising the floor of the mouth, its usefulness as an
indicator of protrusive activity is somewhat questionable. Recent investiga-
tions in our laboratory (A.A. Lowe and B.J. Sessle, *J. dent. Res.* 53 [Special
Issue, 1974] : 201) have revealed that EMG activity of genioglossus (the main
protruder of the tongue) and concommitant tongue protrusion occurs both in
spontaneous and superior laryngeal nerve (SLN)-induced swallows in cats and
monkeys. This genioglossus activity was the first recorded in the swallow synergy, and preceded that of mylohyoid, digastric, and pharyngeal and laryngeal
muscles.

The incidence of SLN-induced swallowing could be increased by mechanical stimulation of canine teeth. This effect is relatively specific since mechanical or electrical stimulation of upper lip and forepaw and auditory stimuli did
not have this facilitatory effect. This may be relevant clinically in relation to
the 'tooth together' swallow pattern which is frequently classified as being
normal, in contrast to the 'tooth apart' swallow.

Jaw position also has a profound influence on genioglossus activity, and
the amount of activity varies in direct accordance with the amount of jaw
opening (A.A. Lowe and B.J. Sessle, *Canad. J. Physiol. Pharmacol.* 51 [1973] :
1009-11). The effect could be reversibly abolished by bilateral infiltration of
local anaesthetic into the region of the temporomandibular joints. We have
also noted that isolated stimulation of joint afferents evokes a reproducible

genioglossus reflex. Alterations in tongue protrusive activity related to changes in the vertical dimension have also been noted clinically (E.P. Harvold, *Am. J. Orthod.* 63 [1973] : 494-508).

Finally, I do not totally agree with the negative reference to myofunctional therapy which inferred that the use of muscle exercises for retraining the tongue are of no clinical use. Some early genioglossus activity often precedes the genioglossus activity associated with swallowing and may indeed be susceptible to training. This area requires much more additional investigation before we can conclusively decide on the validity of using myofunctional therapy as an adjunct to orthodontic treatment.

STOREY I think the mylohyoid is probably participating in a stabilization function. In Møller's records you will notice that the anterior temporal muscle was more active. If the teeth are apart, how is the mandible going to be stabilized? Once the teeth come together, stabilization is achieved without the need for antagonistic muscle effort. Thus activity in the mylohyoid with the teeth apart is not necessarily an indication of tongue protrusion, but rather reflects the need for stabilization.

KAWAMURA When one is looking at muscle activity in the muscles of mastication, one should also consider head position. We have records of swallowing carried out with different positioning of the neck and head, and the muscle activity varies under these circumstances. For example, suprahyoid muscle activity is weak when one swallows tipped up (Y. Kawamura, *Frontiers of Oral Physiology.* Vol. 1. *Physiology of Mastication.* [Basel: Karger, 1974]).

LUND I would like to make a comment about tendon organs. I would be the last person to de-emphasize the importance of tendon organs, because I have just found some, but there are two points that bother me. First, the threshold of tendon organs to active contraction is very low, in most cases less than 1 gm (J.C. Houk et al., *J. Neurophysiol.* 34 [1971]: 1051-65). Therefore tendon organs are presumably firing throughout contraction, and I do not believe that they are suddenly activated to turn it off at a given threshold. Secondly, the switch which occurs from opening to closing can occur without feedback, and one does not have to postulate any peripheral mechanism to cause this (P.G. Dellow and J.P. Lund, *J. Physiol. (Lond.)* 215 [1971]: 1-13).

MATTHEWS There are a number of pauses in motor activity which may not all be caused by the same mechanism. In other parts of the body, Renshaw cells have been implicated, but since masticatory motoneurones lack collaterals, this is unlikely to be the case here. Another possibility would be inhibition from Golgi tendon organs which have been mentioned. A third possibility, which I do not think people have given enough attention to, is that a pause in electrical activity may be due to synchronization of motor units. If a large number of motor units are all active asynchronously at relatively low rates, and then a stimulus is applied which will tend to activate the units and synchronize their firing, there will tend to be an enforced pause following the stimulus as the units return to their previous firing rates. Consequently one does not need any special inhibitory mechanism to create a gap in the recorded response of several units.

SESSLE Yes, there are quite a number of mechanisms capable of causing a silent period in jaw-closing muscle activity and the 'active' inhibitory mechanisms actually involve a whole range of different receptor types (S.-K.J. Yu et al., *Archs oral Biol.* 18 [1973]: 861–70; K. Meier-Ewert et al., *Electroenceph. clin. Neurophysiol.* 36 [1974]: 629–37). We did not indicate that periodontal receptors were the sole cause of inhibition during mastication, although we did find that in our experimental arrangement (*not* mastication) such receptors largely account for the inhibition of jaw-closing muscle activity produced by controlled mechanical stimulation of one tooth (Sessle and Schmitt, 1972). Likewise, peripheral factors affecting lip and tongue activity are not restricted to just one of two sources, as Møller suggests, but are many and varied (e.g. B.J. Sessle and D.J. Kenny, in J.F. Bosma (ed.), *4th Symposium on Oral Sensation and Perception* [Bethesda: D.H.E.W., 1973]).

GOLDBERG As a brief comment with regard to motor control during jaw closing in mastication, which Møller raised, I am not sure that one can assume that gamma drive precedes, or leads, alpha motoneurone activation. I think we have already seen from previous discussions at this symposium that there is evidence for alpha-gamma coactivation in jaw movements.

MØLLER Three points of my report have been especially questioned: lip action during mastication, the electromyogram from the mylohyoid muscle as indicator of tongue action, and the role of the tendon organs in the terminal inhibition of the elevators during mastication. Strong lip action during the opening phase of the chewing stroke (primary activity) is a consistent finding in numerous electromyographic studies of subjects of all ages. Fine wire electrodes have located this activity to the oral sphincter, the orbicularis oris (cf. Fig. 4). Whether the primary activity results in a complete anterior seal or merely prevents the lips from being separated just as much as the jaws (e.g. Australian aborigines) is of little importance. From a neurophysiological point of view the significant finding is that activity causing the lips to approach increases with morphological traits tending to impede lip closure. It is unacceptable to consider the primary activity entirely as a function of social environment. In the foetus, intraoral stimulation may result in lip closure, and I consider the complete or partial seal in children and adults as a reflex initiated at mucosal receptors to prevent food from escaping the oral cavity.

I agree with Lowe that my statements concerning tongue protrusion must be evaluated on the basis of recordings from the intrinsic tongue muscles.

However, the fact that such recordings are not yet available ought not to prevent interpretation of coincidence of early mylohyoid activity and morphological traits tending to impede lip closure (Møller, 1966, Table 40, Fig. 80).
The mylohyoid muscles act strongly when the tongue is pressed against the
palate or protruded. Therefore, I feel quite confident in using its activity as a
certain indirect measure of tongue action, although in principle it acts to raise
the floor of the mouth and stabilize the hyoid bone. Recordings from the
genioglossus may be preferable, but evidence for the lead of this muscle may
not be unanimous (cf. R. Doty and J.F. Bosma, *J. Neurophysiol.* 19 [1956]:
44-60; A.W. Hrycyshyn and J.V. Basmajian, *Am. J. Anat.* 133 [1972]: 333-
40). My recordings during swallowing were obtained with the subject sitting
without head rest. Altering head or body position may affect timing, but not
the intensity of the activity in the suprahyoid muscles (E. Møller et al., *Scand.
J. dent. Res.* 79 [1971]: 483-7; A.W. Hrycyshyn and J.V. Basmajian, 1972).

Lund is correct about the low thresholds of the tendon organs during
active contraction. However, it is this particular fact that gives them a role in
reflex control during natural function instead of acting merely to protect
against extensive overload. The ability of the tendon organs to inhibit the elevators does not imply sudden activation. Their afferent activity increases during contraction until it becomes significant in the total pattern of inhibitory
and facilitatory activity acting on the motoneurones.

Based on statistical coincidence, specific patterns of muscle activity during
mastication and swallowing have been related to morphology and occlusion.
To substitute the mechanical concept of oral function with a neurophysiological one, two tentative mechanisms of biological coherence have been advanced. One couples facial morphology with lip and tongue function by an
exteroceptive mechanism. The other links occlusion with the action of the
elevators through afferent activity (1) from periodontal receptors during
natural circumstances with a facilitating effect (cf. A.J. Thexton, *Brain Res.*
66 [1974]: 425-33), (2) from muscle spindles performing continuous adjust-
ments due to concomitant (no leading!) fusimotor innervation (cf. Vallbo,
J. Physiol. (Lond.) 218 [1971]: 405-31), and (3) from tendon organs responsible for the final inhibition. Even if one of the mechanisms just mentioned
may have to be replaced (cf. G. Goodwin and E. Luchei, *J. Neurophysiol.* 37
[1974]: 967-81), the extensive variation of muscle activity during mastication points strongly to a dominating peripheral mechanism of control. Central
control calls for extensive study because it has more value as a processer than
as an independent mechanism.

Oral-facial sensation in the control of mastication and voluntary movements of the jaw

J.P. LUND

ROLE IN THE GENERATION OF THE
BASIC MASTICATORY PATTERN

The coordination and alternation of mastication were for many years attributed to the alternate activation of the jaw-opening reflex and jaw-closing
myotatic reflex (Sherrington, 1917; Rioch, 1934). However, it has now been
definitely established that the basic movements are patterned within the brain
stem without proprioceptive feedback (Lund and Dellow, 1969, 1973; Sumi,
1970 a,b; Dellow and Lund, 1971). However, the brain stem masticatory pattern generator, which can be driven by electrical stimulation of various forebrain and midbrain structures (for details see Magoun, Ranson, and Fisher,
1933; Kawamura and Tsukamoto, 1960; Sumi, 1969; Lund and Dellow,
1971), can also be excited from the oral cavity of paralyzed, decerebrate animals (Lund and Dellow, 1973). The central and peripheral stimuli can be
shown to sum (Lund and Dellow, 1973, Fig. 2a), presumably in the pattern
generator.

Strong excitatory or inhibitory coupling is apparently needed to account
for the regular appearance of synchronized bursts in many neurones (Wilson
and Waldron, 1968). Trigeminal and hypoglossal motoneurones probably do
not have the collaterals required for coupling (Ramón y Cajal, 1909). Furthermore, they are not affected by antidromic stimulation of adjacent cells (Porter,
1965; Kidokoro et al., 1968). All available evidence indicates that the pattern
of mastication is generated by a pool of interneurones in the brain stem.

The nature of peripheral stimuli which will cause mastication is not well
understood but is apparently not proprioceptive. In some other systems, proprioceptive feedback is not necessary for the genesis of rhythmic movements,
but it does increase the frequency of the output (Wilson and Wyman, 1965).
When masticatory activity is produced by electrical stimulation of the corti-
cobulbar tracts in rabbits with empty mouths, the form of the input-output

relation curve (Dellow and Lund, 1971, Fig. 7) is unchanged after paralysis. This suggests that proprioceptive feedback from muscle receptors and the temporomandibular joints (TMJ) has little influence on the frequency output of the masticatory pattern generator.

Bremer (1923) produced rhythmical mastication in decerebrate rabbits by rubbing the corners of the mouth; it can also be induced by blowing up a small balloon between the tongue and hard palate (Lund and Dellow, 1973). Opening the jaw by hand is ineffective, so it was assumed that stimulation of oral tactile and pressure receptors caused the response. Since rhythmic bursts of activity continued in the hypoglossal nerves of paralyzed rabbits for more than 20 sec during the balloon inflation (Lund and Dellow, 1973, Fig. 1c), the receptors involved are apparently slowly adapting.

It is well known that the rate of mastication is, to a large extent, governed by the texture of food. In man, soft foods are eaten slowly and hard foods rapidly (e.g. Steiner, Michman, and Litman, 1974). Presently it is not known if a frequency change during mastication results from an increase in tactile and pressure receptor input. However, the output of the pattern generator is proportional to the rate and intensity of electrical stimulation of the forebrain, at least over a narrow range of input parameters (Sumi, 1970b, Fig. 4; Dellow and Lund, 1971, Fig. 6). Thus, it is reasonable to suppose that the output is modulated by the temporal and spatial characteristics of the peripheral input.

INTERACTION OF PERIPHERAL STIMULI WITH THE BASIC MASTICATORY PATTERN

Non-specific suppression

Rectal distention, paw pinching, and undoubtedly other noxious stimuli depress centrally elicited mastication in the anaesthetized or decerebrate rabbit (Lund and Dellow, 1969, 1973). Segmental reflexes seem to be similarly depressed. Kubota, Kidokoro, and Suzuki (1968) found that stimulation of the superficial radial nerve in the cat suppressed both flexor and extensor reflexes along the whole length of the neuraxis. IPSPs were recorded concurrently in lumbar flexor and extensor motoneurones and in motoneurones of the jaw-closing muscles. It is probable that this general inhibition of reflexes and mastication is brought about by the brain stem reticular formation (Kubota et al., 1968; Sumi, 1971).

The first few masticatory cycles which follow the removal of an inhibitory stimulus often occur at a faster rate than that observed before inhibition. As previously stated, it appears that the motoneurones receive an input which has already been patterned into alternating bursts by other elements within the brain stem. Although motoneuronal excitability may be raised during the period immediately following an ipsp (Coombs, Curtis, and Eccles, 1959), possibly increasing the number of spikes/burst, this can hardly be expected to change the rate at which the bursts are generated. This rebound acceleration of the chewing rate is, therefore, indirect evidence that inhibition must also take place at the level of the masticatory pattern generator.

Suppression by oral-facial afferents

It is possible that oral-facial inputs which are presumably noxious (see paper by Greenwood and Sessle, this volume) may suppress mastication by acting on motoneurones and on the pattern generator (Sumi, 1970b). The action of such inputs at the motoneuronal level is well documented (see papers by Greenwood and Sessle, and by Goldberg, this volume). Suppression can be achieved through segmental reflexes as well as by longer pathways involving the reticular formation (Sumino, 1971) or cortex (Lund and Sessle, 1974). Other inputs from all the various oral, facial, laryngeal, and pharyngeal structures which have been shown to influence excitability of motoneurones (e.g. Schmitt, Yu, and Sessle, 1973) must similarly modify the final output of the system, as discussed in the first workshop report. Fundamental but complex activities such as swallowing interrupt cortically evoked chewing (Sumi, 1969, 1970a). However, the levels at which this suppression occurs have not yet been delineated.

Proprioceptive feedback

Experiments on the influence of tmj afferents on active movements have not been reported. Kawamura and Majima (1964) demonstrated that the firing of masseteric motoneurones were depressed by jaw closure and activated by jaw opening. The converse relation was observed for digastric motoneurones.

The influence of periodontal pressoreceptors on jaw-closing motoneurones has been discussed already by other participants. However, mention will be made of the modification of the basic masticatory pattern caused by a specific type of stimulation of these receptors. Prolonged pressure applied to the incisor tooth of rabbits causes the mandible to swing to the opposite side of the mouth (Lund and Dellow, 1971, Fig. 3; Lund, McLachlan, and Dellow, 1971). If light pressure is applied during stimulus-evoked mastication in decerebrate rabbits, the movements which were previously made only in the vertical plane now include a swing to the contralateral side during closure. Other responses whose character depends on the intensity, duration, or spatial distribution of the stimulus (Thexton, 1973) may modify mastication. This might occur at the motoneurone or by modification of the pattern by which motoneurone groups are sequentially activated.

Humans deprived of periodontal input by local anaesthesia are unable to exert their previously determined maximal biting force (Lund and Lamarre, 1973, Fig. 2). These data and other results obtained from cortical recording with microelectrodes in chronic monkeys, have prompted the suggestion that periodontal receptors are the sensors in a force-control system for voluntary jaw closure (Lund and Lamarre, 1973, 1974a). Houk, Singer, and Goldman (1970) and Stein (1974) have described how Golgi tendon organs, which have many analogies with periodontal receptors, could act in a negative-feedback, tension-control, system. However, nothing is known about the importance of tendon organ afferents in the control of jaw movements; in fact, except for a single sentence in Szentagothai's (1948) paper, such receptors have never been conclusively described in jaw muscles. Tendon organs have recently been found in the jaw-closing muscles of newborn kittens and in monkey masseter, temporalis, and digastric muscles (Lund, Touloumis, Patry, Richmond, and Lamarre, unpublished observations). Their importance remains to be evaluated.

Recordings have been made (Matsunami and Kubota, 1972; Cody and Taylor, 1973; Taylor and Cody, 1974) from jaw-closing muscle spindle primary afferents within the trigeminal mesencephalic nucleus of awake cats and monkeys. No neuronal discharges precede EMG activity in the muscles of origin and therefore the 'length-follow-up servo' hypothesis originally proposed by Merton (1953) and used by Murphy (1967) to explain the control of jaw muscles, is not valid. However, firing of both primary and secondary afferents continues during active jaw closure. This is in contrast to the cessation of firing brought about by passive closure (Taylor and Davey, 1968). As in the case of movements analyzed to date, alpha-gamma coactivation presumably occurs during jaw closure (Matthews, 1972).

Recent experiments demonstrate the participation of spindle afferents of the jaw-closing muscles in load compensation (Lund and Lamarre, 1974b). In these studies, human subjects moved a lever fixed to the spindle of a torque motor with their lower jaws while the upper teeth rested on a fixed bar (Fig. 1). Subjects were trained to close their jaw at constant velocity, and in randomly selected trials torque pulses were applied either to oppose or aid the movement.

EMG activity in the masseter and temporalis muscles increased abruptly 5-10 msec (mean 7.2 msec) after loading began, even if the load was insufficient to stretch the muscles. This latency was essentially the same as that of the jaw-jerk reflex. The mandible began to rise again 6-10 msec after the peak EMG response and, if the load was removed, its velocity exceeded the control

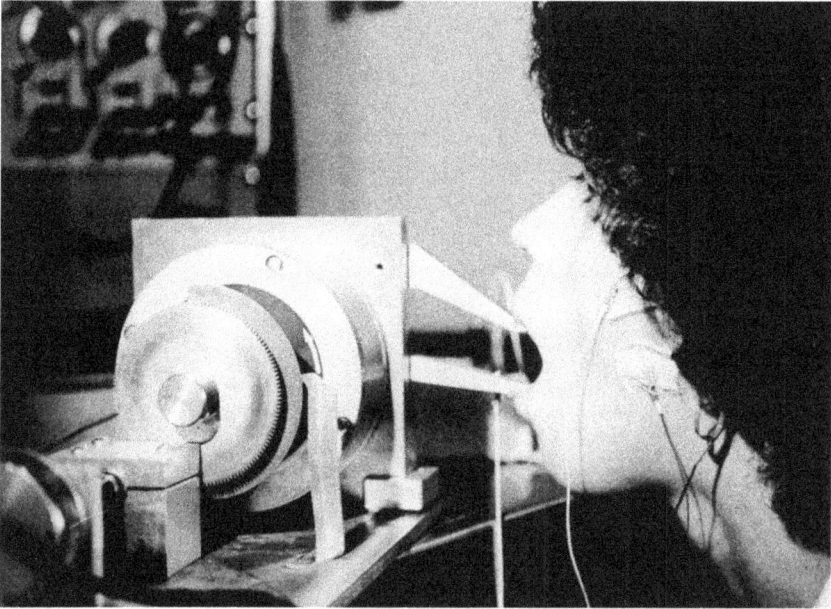

FIGURE 1   Subject and experimental apparatus. Biting on the lever turns the spindle of the torque motor, which is connected by a system of gears to the potentiometer at the far left. The active EMG electrode is placed over the masseter and a reference electrode over the zygoma.

rate. If the subject was instructed to resist the pulse when it arrived, the early monosynaptic response and the velocity of movement were increased. In addition, a late response was seen at a latency equal to that of the early voluntary activity which followed stimulation of the mouth (Fig. 2). If the jaw-closing muscles were unloaded, then the level of EMG activity fell after a delay of 7–16 msec. This strongly suggests that a large part of the input to the alpha motoneurones must be arriving via the Ia afferents. In contrast, the digastric muscles, which according to the principle of reciprocal inhibition should restrain an unexpected release of the jaw-closing muscles, only became active after 24 msec.

None of these responses were reduced by the infiltration of local anaesthetic about the roots of the teeth which gripped the apparatus. In fact, the height of the monosynaptic response was significantly increased by 80 per cent after local anaesthesia.

Studies of the thumb and intercostal muscles of humans have shown that the monosynaptic stretch reflex does not provide load compensation (Sears,

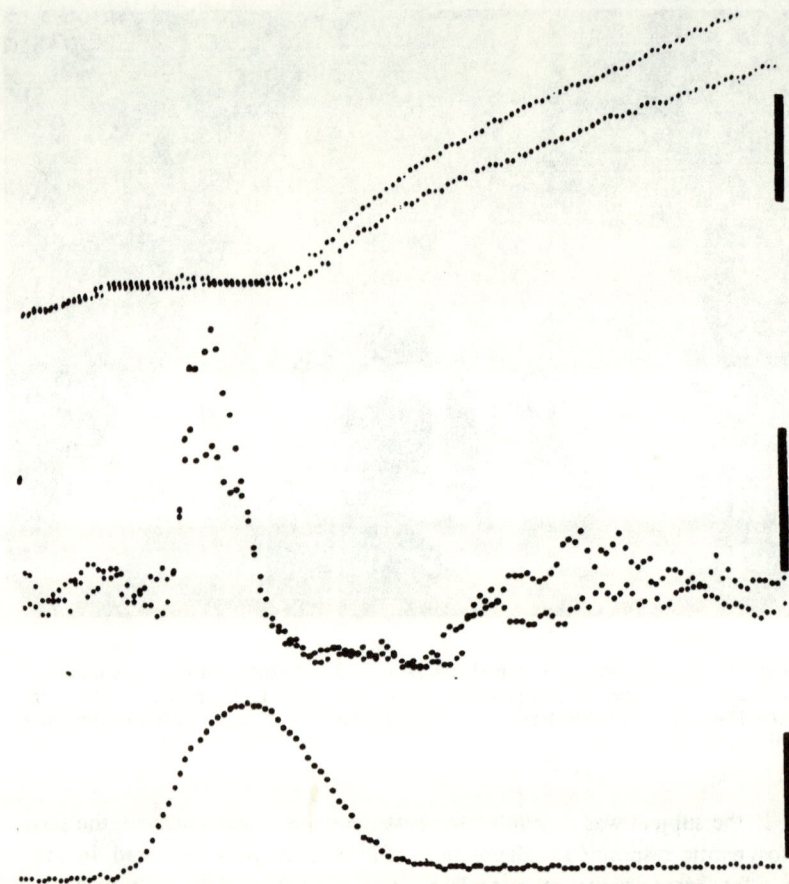

FIGURE 2 Photograph from the oscilloscope screen of the output of the signal aver-
ager. The displacement (upper trace) and integrated EMG (middle trace) are averaged
over 16 trials. The lower trace shows force measurements made when the levers were
clamped together. Two series of trials were superimposed: in the first, the subject was
told not to resist and, in the second, he was told to resist the loading pulse. Bin width: 1
msec (total display, 127 msec). Calibration: 2 mm; 100 μV; 200 gm.

1973: Merton, 1974). This compensation is provided by a rapid cortical loop
and a later voluntary response. Monosynaptic load compensation may provide
a more efficient mechanism in the masticatory system because the resistance
to closure is constantly and rapidly changing. Food is not of uniform texture
and mastication itself alters the resistance to crushing and penetration. By
using a servo-assistance system (Stein, 1974), the breakage of a peanut during

crushing would be followed, with monosynaptic latency, by a rapid fall in alpha motoneurone output, while a seed inside a slice of tomato could be crushed by monosynaptic augmentation of alpha motoneurone output.

ACKNOWLEDGMENTS

The author is a Scholar of the Canadian Medical Research Council and its continuing support is gratefully acknowledged. Photographic illustrations were prepared by Messrs E. Rupnik, R. Péloquin and D. Cyr. Technical assistance was ably provided by Mr R. Bouchoux. Drs Y. Lamarre and E. Puil kindly read and criticized earlier drafts of this manuscript.

REFERENCES

Bremer, F. 1923. Physiologie nerveuse de la mastication chez le chat et le lapin. *Archs int. Physiol.* 21: 308–52

Cody, F.W.J., and Taylor, A. 1973. The behaviour of spindles in the jaw-closing muscles during eating and drinking in the cat. *J. Physiol. (Lond.)* 231: 49–50P

Coombs, J.J., Curtis, D.R., and Eccles, J.C. 1959. The electrical constants of the motoneurone membrane. *J. Physiol. (Lond.)* 145: 505–28

Dellow, P.G., and Lund, J.P. 1971. Evidence for central timing of rhythmical mastication. *J. Physiol. (Lond.)* 215: 1–13

Houk, J., Singer, J.J., and Goldman, M.R. 1970. An evaluation of length and force feedback in decerebrate cats. *J. Neurophysiol.* 33: 784–811

Kawamura, Y., and Majima, T. 1964. Temporomandibular joint's sensory mechanisms controlling activities of jaw muscles. *J. dent. Res.* 43: 150

Kawamura, Y., and Tsukamoto, S. 1960. Analysis of jaw movements from the cortical jaw motor area and amygdala. *Jap. J. Physiol.* 10: 471–88

Kidokoro, Y., Kubota, K., Shuto, S., and Sumino, R. 1968. Reflex organization of cat masticatory muscles. *J. Neurophysiol.* 31: 695–708

Kubota, K., Kidokoro, Y., and Suzuki, J. 1968. Postsynaptic inhibitions of trigeminal and lumbar motoneurones from the superfacial radial nerve in the cat. *Jap. J. Physiol.* 18: 198–215

Lund, J.P., and Dellow, P.G. 1969. Evidence for a central rhythmical drive of jaw muscles. *Canada Physiol.* 1: 50

– 1971. The influence of interactive stimuli on rhythmical masticatory movements in rabbits. *Archs oral Biol.* 16: 215–23

– 1973. Rhythmical masticatory activity of hypoglossal motoneurons responding to an oral stimulus. *Exp. Neurol.* 40: 223–46

Lund, J.P., and Lamarre, Y. 1973. The importance of positive feedback from periodontal pressoreceptors during voluntary isometric contraction of jaw closing muscles in man. *J. biol. bucc.* 1: 345–51

— 1974a. Activity of neurons in the lower precentral cortex during voluntary and rhythmical jaw movements in the monkey. *Exp. Brain Res.* 19: 282–99

— 1974b. Monosynaptic load compensation in human jaw muscles. *Proc. Canad. Fed. Biol. Soc.* 17: 102

Lund, J.P., McLachlan, R.S., and Dellow, P.G. 1971. A lateral jaw movement reflex. *Exp. Neurol.* 31: 189–99

Lund, J.P., and Sessle, B.J. 1974. Oral-facial and jaw muscle afferent projections to neurones in cat frontal cortex. *Exp. Neurol.* 45: 314–31

Magoun, H.W., Ranson, S.W., and Fisher, C. 1933. Cortico-fugal pathways for mastication, lapping and other motor functions in the cat. *Archs Neurol. Psychiat.* 30: 292–308

Matsunami, K., and Kubota, K. 1972. Muscle afferents of trigeminal mesencephalic tract nucleus and mastication in chronic monkeys. *Jap. J. Physiol.* 22: 545–55

Matthews, P.B.C. 1972. *Mammalian Muscle Receptors and Their Central Actions.* London: Arnold

Merton, P.A. 1953. Speculations on the servo control of movement. In G.E. Wolstenholme (ed.), *The Spinal Cord.* London: Churchill

— 1974. The properties of the human muscle servo. *Brain Res.* 71: 475–8

Murphy, T.R. 1967. Shortening/inhibition of prime movers. A safety factor in mastication. *Brit. dent. J.* 123: 578–84

Porter, R. 1965. Synaptic potentials in hypoglossal motoneurones. *J. Physiol. (Lond.)* 180: 209–24

Ramón y Cajal, S. 1909. *Histologie du Système Nerveux de l'Homme et des Vertébrés.* Paris: Maloine

Rioch, J.M. 1934. Neural mechanisms of mastication. *Am. J. Physiol.* 108: 168–76

Schmitt, A., Yu, S.-K.J., and Sessle, B.J. 1973. Excitatory and inhibitory influences from laryngeal and orofacial areas on tongue position in the cat. *Archs oral Biol.* 18: 1121–30

Sears, T.A. 1973. Servo control of the intercostal muscles. In J.E. Desmedt (ed.), *New Developments in Electromyography and Clinical Neurophysiology.* Vol. 3. Basel: Karger

Sherrington, C.S. 1917. Reflexes elicitable in the cat from pinna, vibrissae and jaws. *J. Physiol. (Lond.)* 51: 404–31

Stein, R.B. 1974. Peripheral control of movement. *Physiol. Rev.* 54: 215–43

Steiner, J.E., Michman, J., and Litman, A. 1974. Time sequence of the activity of the temporal and masseter muscles in healthy young human adults
during habitual chewing of different test foods. *Archs oral Biol.* 19: 29–34

Sumi, T. 1969. Some properties of cortically-evoked swallowing and chewing
in rabbits. *Brain Res.* 15: 107–20

– 1970a. Activity in single hypoglossal fibers during cortically induced
swallowing and chewing in rabbits. *Pflügers Arch.* 314: 329–46

– 1970b. Changes of hypoglossal nerve activity during inhibition of chewing
and swallowing by lingual nerve stimulation. *Pflügers Arch.* 317: 303–9

– 1971. Modification of cortically evoked rhythmical chewing and swallowing from midbrain and pons. *Jap. J. Physiol.* 21: 489–506

Sumino, R. 1971. Central neural pathways involved in the jaw opening reflex
in the cat. In R. Dubner and Y. Kawamura (eds.), *Oral-Facial Sensory and
Motor Mechanisms.* New York: Appleton-Century-Crofts

Szentagothai, J. 1948. Anatomical considerations of monosynaptic reflex
arcs. *J. Neurophysiol.* 11: 445–54

Taylor, A., and Cody, F.W.F. 1974. Jaw muscle spindle activity in the cat
during normal movements of eating and drinking. *Brain Res.* 71: 523–30

Taylor, A., and Davey, M.R. 1968. Behaviour of the jaw muscle stretch receptors during active and passive movements in cats. *Nature* 220: 301–2

Thexton, A.J. 1973. Oral reflexes elicited by mechanical stimulation of
palatal mucosa in the cat. *Archs oral Biol.* 18: 971–80

Wilson, D.M., and Waldron, I. 1968. Models for the generation of the motor
output pattern in flying locusts. *Proc. Instn. elect. Engrs.* 56: 1058–64

Wilson, D.M., and Wyman, R.J. 1965. Motor output patterns during random
and rhythmic stimulation of locust thoracic ganglia. *Biophys. J.* 5: 121–43

DISCUSSION

SESSLE Dr Lund, it would seem that periodontal receptors are not responsible for the effects that you report. In studies on the thumb, which were
fairly similar to your work (C.D. Marsden et al., *Nature* 238 [1972]: 140-3),
anaesthetizing around the wrist, produced a facilitatory effect. I believe joint
or cutaneous receptors were implicated, and I wondered whether these receptors might play a part in your system.

MATTHEWS I thought those experiments implicated only cutaneous receptors. They were asking subjects to follow guide signals, and examined the response in the muscles in the forearm following a sudden increase in resistance
to movement. The local anaesthetic did not affect muscle receptors, but the

cutaneous receptors would have been anaesthetized. I believe they showed the cutaneous receptors were involved in the response and this suggests that some positive feedback may have been occurring in the normal response.

LUND   They suggested that the cutaneous input is very important for regulation of the gain of the cortical servo-loop, but I have not seen any good evidence that shows that this cortical loop relies upon spindle input. It could just as well rely on cutaneous input, the gain of the cutaneous input being regulated by the spindle input.

KUBOTA   Have you tried looking at the jaw-opening muscles?

LUND   Yes, but we did not see an early response. We have not tried to see whether we could increase it by learning. I do not think the jaw-opening muscles can be primarily implicated in the opposition to increased speed of jaw closure during unloading. I think this has to come by inhibition of the jaw-closing muscles.

THOMAS   You feel that you had sufficient anaesthesia of the periodontal ligament?

LUND   Well, we had enough to produce an effect, in this case an increase in the monosynaptic component.

MATTHEWS   This is interesting, because we have been looking recently at the effect of mechanical stimulation of the teeth on the monosynaptic reflex evoked by brief opening movements in decerebrate cats. We have found that local anaesthetic infiltrated around the canine region would often be followed by potentiation of the monosynaptic response. Incidentally, one has to be careful not to give toxic doses of local anaesthesia to the animals under these circumstances. The usual 2 ml cartridge of lignocaine (40 mg) is way above the minimum dose (1 mg/kg) that begins to depress cortical activity in the cat (C.G. Bernard et al., *Archs int. Pharmacodyn. Ther.* 108 [1956] : 392–419).

LOWE   Would you comment on the methods employed in your previous studies to identify the hypoglossal nucleus and the criteria used to differentiate the responses you recorded from phasic respiratory discharges? Do the records correlate with masticatory movements?

LUND   Identification was done on histological grounds, not by electrical stimulation. The responses are not respiratory, because the respiratory rhythm is much slower than these, and one can often see this in background activity. In the unanaesthetized animal, they are also in phase with masticatory activity.

SESSLE   Have you carried out any experiments to test the functional role of what appear to be tendon organs?

LUND   No, we have not yet gone that far. They are not as numerous as spindles; so far we think about half the number for the masseter muscle. I assume that if they are there in large enough numbers, they are functional. They always appear to be associated with spindles in the masseter and temporalis muscles.

SESSLE   The reason I asked about function is that in the paper by Kidokoro et al. (1968) that you cite, no evidence of Group Ib afferent effects on cat masseter motoneurones was observed with electrical stimulation. Perhaps with electrical stimulation of masseter nerve a central interaction between Ia and Ib afferents occurs, and the excitation masks any Ib inhibition.

LUND   I can only say that from the work on neck muscles, which have more spindles/gm than other muscles, that one cannot obtain a monosynaptic reflex even with electrical stimulation (V.C. Abrahams et al., *Brain Res.* 92 [1975]: 130-1). In other words just because they are there, it does not mean that they are projecting back onto the same motoneurones.

SESSLE   It would also be interesting to see whether tendon organs are in the pterygoid muscles as well.

LUND   Since the Golgi tendon organs must be firing off every time the muscles contract, they may be affecting far more than their own motoneurones. Moreover, they could have a strong influence on cortical neurones, and this could be far more important than their local influence.

GOLDBERG   During cortical stimulation, what is the implication of having, for example, a constant output frequency of, say, 2/sec in one case versus 4/sec in another? In other words the pattern is the same, but the output frequency changes.

LUND   I do not know how profitable it would be to go into this. One could propose all sorts of neuronal models to achieve this effect, but we do not really know how to account for it. All we can say is that it is a property of the brain stem circuitry. It does saturate however.

STOREY   My question concerns the equivalent of the unloading situation, where you are recording from the digastric. You have shown that inhibition occurs in the levators. You will agree with me that the lateral pterygoid is a depressor, and that it is necessary that the lateral pterygoid and digastric muscles function in the same way. We know that in volitional movements, they do not behave in the same way. Do you think, before you dismiss the possibility, that the lateral pterygoid is doing the same as the digastric?

LUND   I agree that one cannot make any assumptions.

DUBNER   In your loading experiments, are you really sure you are not producing any stretch of the spindles?

LUND   No, but the most likely effect is that we are getting spindle unloading because of the compliance of the muscle insertions. When we set up the experiment, we adjust the appliance so that there is no muscle stretch.

MATTHEWS   What range of dynamic loadings did you use in this work?

LUND   The loads were of the order of 100-400 gm.

MATTHEWS These are pretty small in terms of masticatory loads. If you increased the load you might bring in, for example, periodontal influences.

KUBOTA The idea that a long descending reflex through the motor cortex from the muscle spindle may be important for the control of movement is not a popular hypothesis at present (C.G. Phillips et al., *J. Physiol. (Lond.)* 217 [1971] : 419–46; H.L. Teuber, *Brain Res.* 71 [1974] : 533–68). Evidence is not available which shows any influence of cortical cells on the descending reflex path.

LUND There have been recordings made (E. Evarts, *Science* 197 [1972] : 501–3) of pyramidal tract cells during these reflexes; they respond as one would expect of neurones with this function.

KUBOTA These are cutaneous inputs.

LUND Yes, I do not think that it has been established that this is a spindle loop, although we now have evidence for a Group I afferent projection from jaw-closing muscles to frontal cortex of cat (Lund and Sessle, 1974).

Chairman's Summary

A.G. HANNAM

In this session we have discussed some of the patterns of muscle activity to be expected during mastication and swallowing, and we have explored some of the mechanisms which may be involved in the development of these patterns, in particular those associated with chewing. The role of afferent feedback from the oral area has been emphasized, not only with regard to its contribution at the level of the brain stem and the reflex events which can be demonstrated as a result, but also in terms of the afferent contribution at the suprasegmental level, and the effect this has in modifying the direction and force of voluntary jaw movements. We have seen an expressed interest in the role of the Golgi tendon organ, and a desire to determine just where these afferents project and what they actually do in function. We have reaffirmed the inhibitory and excitatory influence of periodontal afferent neurones on jaw-elevator muscles, and then speculated upon their influence on higher centres, for example the cortex, raising the intriguing proposition that they may be involved in a positive-feedback loop at this level. We have discussed the various contribution to the silent pause in elevator muscle activity which occurs on tooth contact, and appear to be agreed that many inputs can cause inhibition of this kind, for example, periodontal ligament afferents, muscle spindle afferents, and even auditory nerve afferents. Finally, we have seen some very interesting experimental data which would suggest the coactivation of alpha and gamma motoneurones in the jaw-closing muscles during voluntary clenching tasks. We are still a long way from understanding how neural mechanisms above the brain stem operate to create the plasticity which characterizes normal mastication, but it is encouraging to find more and more attention diverted away from the brain stem, which seems to have claimed so much of our time over the last few years.

It is clear that we must be careful to adjust our concepts of normal muscle function as more data becomes available. We cannot continue to use the simplistic definitions of agonist and antagonist masticatory muscle actions given in conventional anatomical texts, because the activity of these muscles often overlaps, or is concurrent, in function. Here, the actions of the lateral pterygoid and digastric muscles are a good example. Moreover, in the normal state, reciprocal arrangements between muscles of the right and the left sides may prove to be very significant in terms of the control of jaw movements. There seems to be a tendency for us to think in up and down terms rather than in side to side terms, a phenomenon due, perhaps, to the numbers of experiments we have carried out on cats.

In this section, we have also seen the value of pattern analysis of the activity of various muscles during mastication and swallowing, both as a basic research tool to further our understanding of normal behaviour, and as a means of detecting pathology. In addition, we have been alerted to the need for recording from specific muscles in order to define coordinated functions with any reliability. Particular emphasis has been placed on the muscles of the face and lips, and the separate actions of the genioglossus and mylohyoid muscles during swallowing.

In conclusion, it seems that in the future we shall probably be in a better position to correlate the results of chronic animal experiments with those of humans in normal function, especially in the field of primate research. This increasing ability to define muscle function with equal sensitivity in both experimental environments can only be to our advantage.

SECTION FIVE

Workshop group reports

How are mastication and swallowing programmed and regulated?

B.J. SESSLE

This report summarizes the highlights of the deliberations of the first work-shop group comprising L.J. Goldberg, K. Kubota, J.P. Lund, B. Matthews, and B.J. Sessle (Chairman), and of the lively discussion that followed the presentation of their answer to the question posed. The report represents collective impressions where possible, and is not an exhaustive literature review on the topic (for review, see Doty, 1968; Kawamura, 1974; and previous papers in this volume). For ease of presentation, swallowing and mastication, within the context of the question, will for the most part be considered separately.

SWALLOWING

As pointed out earlier in this symposium by Storey, swallowing must be considered as an airway protective reflex in addition to its role in alimentary function. Thus much discussion was spent on defining what is meant by 'swallowing.' It appears to occur very early in foetal life (Humphrey, 1970; Bradley and Mistretta, 1973) and was considered to represent an innate primary pattern of coordinated oral-facial muscle activity. Attention was drawn especially to the oral and pharyngeal phases of swallowing, and there are a number of muscles which must be considered as essential in this pattern. These are activated in an all-or-none fashion in a close and reproducible sequence of excitation and inhibition (e.g. Doty and Bosma, 1956). Species and age variations exist as to the muscles involved, but overall, the essential muscles are those of the tongue, pharynx, and larynx (Doty, 1968). The workshop group did not include muscles such as those innervated by the trigeminal nerve since these may or may not be active in swallowing in a particular species. Not all participants, however, agreed with this definition, particularly in view of the criteria used by the workshop group in defining mastication (see below).

Swallowing may be initiated reflexly or voluntarily; once initiated, the event is self-propagating. The voluntary command might be thought of as causing a 'gate' to open in the brain that allows food, saliva, etc. to trigger the event reflexly. There is a maximum rate at which one can swallow, so it appears that the central neural mechanisms are refractory for long periods. Of course, the initiation is dependent upon peripheral conditions. For example, the difficulty of swallowing with a dry mouth and with an open bite is well known. Sensory information from the periodontium appears to facilitate the initiation of swallowing (Lowe and Sessle, 1974). The importance of this periodontal input might conceivably be reflected in the difficulty experienced in swallowing by patients with open bites, in the constancy of the number of chewing strokes before the occurrence of a swallow (Yurkstas, 1965), and in determining the actual occurrence of the swallow (Sessle and Storey, 1972) as Goldberg has mentioned in his presentation at this symposium.

Attention was again drawn to our present uncertainty regarding characteristics of the adequate stimulus for swallowing. For example, what are the factors that determine whether a particular peripheral stimulus initiates swallowing or gagging or coughing? This uncertainty has been discussed in Storey's paper (this volume) and Sessle pointed out that receptors in the same regions from which these events are elicited are also involved in the initiation of other, more elementary, reflex activity in many of the muscles associated with swallowing (see Doty, 1968). These stimuli can also evoke in many of these muscles a considerable amount of what might be termed 'pre-swallowing' activity, which does not necessarily carry through to a swallow. In view of such reflex and abortive-type activity, careful attention must be paid in studies of swallowing in humans and in animals that what one is monitoring is indeed swallowing.

Peripheral feedback

Although peripheral input may be important in the initiation of swallowing, it was felt that there was a considerable amount of evidence (e.g. with nerve sectioning or muscle paralysis) to indicate that the event, once initiated, is not susceptible to sensory feedback. However, experiments apparently have not been carried out to establish, definitively, that the timing and magnitude of activity of the individual muscles involved are not susceptible to peripheral feedback. Goldberg drew attention to citations in his paper (this volume) of exceptions with respect to the role of feedback in swallowing, and of the work of Sessle and Storey (1972) who suggested that sensory influences from the periodontium may hold the swallow in abeyance. Sessle pointed out, however, that he and Storey had also suggested that the negative influence demonstrated by them may be involved in limiting further sensory input into the brain stem which could upset the ongoing neural synergistic events after a swallow is initiated. A somewhat similar concept may apply for sensory input and presynaptic inhibition in invertebrate patterned, sequential activities (e.g. Kennedy, Calabrese, and Wine, 1974) and Sessle has noted (unpublished observations) that the elicitation of oral-facial reflex activity is markedly impaired once a swallow has been initiated in cat and monkey. Perhaps the 30/sec optimum stimulation rate of the superior laryngeal nerve for eliciting swallowing may be a reflection of the peak effect (30-40 msec) of presynaptic depolarization and inhibition in the solitary tract nucleus (Sessle and Storey, 1972; Sessle, 1973).

If the basic swallowing act is a fundamental and obligate reflex, one might not expect it to be modifiable by training. But again exceptions occur (e.g. the champion beer guzzler: see Doty, 1968). Associated movements, such as those occurring in preswallow activities, may, however, be susceptible to modification. Such considerations are, of course, important clinically, for example in tongue thrusting, and the third workshop group report enlarges on this aspect. Storey however made the point at this stage, with respect to learning and swallowing, that Sumi (1975) has recently noted changes in swallowing as a result of neuromuscular blockade in immature animals. This preliminary evidence is an indication of perhaps a learning aspect to swallowing.

Central neural elements

Experiments carried out in animals suggest that an area in the caudal brain stem is implicated in the genesis of the complex swallow pattern in the form of a temporal sequence of muscle activity (Doty, Richmond, and Storey, 1967; Sumi, 1971). This area is probably in the brain stem reticular formation, although Sessle mentioned Jean's view (1972) that neurones in the solitary tract nucleus may also be involved. The possibility was raised that there are command cells capable of driving the motoneurones in their stereotyped pattern of activity. Comparison was made with the central oscillator neurones found in invertebrate systems and associated with feeding behaviour, walking, swimming, insect flight, etc. (e.g. Kater and Rowell, 1973). It is possible that the command cells responsible for swallowing could be non-spiking neurones with a rhythmic, oscillating, membrane potential similar to those seen in invertebrates. Some trepidation was expressed in trying to record from such neurones in mammals.

It was felt that these neurones could be excited by peripheral stimulation and also be susceptible to higher centre input. For example, cortical stimulation can elicit swallowing even in the paralyzed animal, which would suggest that the higher centre input can bypass the reflex input, and activate the command cell directly. However, there was some question about this, and uncertainty was expressed as to whether any work had been carried out in the de-afferented animal to show that cortical stimulation could still elicit swallow-ing. In other words, is the cortical command dependent upon at least some sensory information (e.g. saliva) coming in from the larynx and pharynx?

Because of its innate nature, the basic muscle pattern of swallowing should be preserved during changes in the central state, for example in sleep. This has been borne out experimentally, although the rate of swallowing is profoundly decreased during sleep. However, this may simply be a reflection of decreased salivary flow, and needs testing. In view of the role of swallowing in airway protection, such mechanisms may be important in conditions such as the Sudden Infant (Crib) Death Syndrome, which has a strong relationship with sleep and which has been discussed in Storey's paper (this volume). Moreover, the high incidence of choking deaths in humans, and its possible causal relationship to alcohol consumption with concomitant central depression, emphasizes the clinical significance of further studies in this area.

MASTICATION

Considerable discussion arose as a result of the workshop group's attempt at defining mastication. It was particularly edifying to this writer to note that a group of eminent clinical and basic scientists working in the field of mastication could not reach a clear understanding or agreement on what was meant by the term! The workshop group viewed mastication as an all-encompassing behaviour pattern that consists of a basic primary pattern of muscle activity upon which is superimposed reflex and higher centre feedbacks. Since mastication is necessary for the breakdown of foodstuffs and their mixing with saliva, processes (e.g. chemical, enzymatic) other than neuromuscular events might be viewed as part of the overall masticatory act.

In contrast to their definition of swallowing as being an innate, obligate, and reproducible event, mastication was considered by the workshop group to consist of a series of sequences of muscle contractions and relaxations, each cycle in the series not necessarily being identical. Matthews stressed the group's view of mastication as being a variable, sequenced pattern of movements which is therefore beyond a simple definition. However, other participants, notably Dubner, Greenwood, and Thomas, took exception to this view. They felt that, if the workshop group considered the 'extraneous' oral-facial activities that may or may not take place in chewing as still part of mastication, then the group had applied too rigid a classification for swallowing as an automated, innate, sequential pattern of muscle activities. For example, 'preswallow' muscle activities should then be considered as part of swallowing. For the sake of consistency and clarity, they argued that the 'masticatory'

analogue of the innate pattern earlier defined as swallowing is the cyclic movements of jaw-opening and jaw-closing.

Goldberg felt strongly that mastication has features quite distinct from
swallowing. He emphasized the workshop group's feeling that the preparatory
phases, such as positioning the food prior to swallowing, are extraneous to
the obligatory swallow. He felt that mastication, in contrast, has no element
of an obligate beginning and end pattern of muscle activity that characterizes
swallowing. He also pointed out the dissociation between swallowing and
mastication in the decerebrate cat, which can swallow but cannot chew in the
full meaning of the word. The need for descending suprasegmental systems,
probably for the crushing aspects of mastication, is thus indicated.

Irrespective of whether one defines mastication in terms of simple cyclical
jaw and tongue movements or as a more complex and variable pattern of muscle activity, the cyclic movement pattern can be readily elicited experimentally. This pattern could be considered to be the important element of the
masticatory act, providing the fundamental framework upon which more
complex patterns are based (Kawamura stressed that species variations of
course occur as to the actual muscle groups involved). There is some similarity
in thinking here with the locomotor patterns involved in walking, but it is significant that uncertainty and controversy still exist as to the genesis of locomotion and the relative importance of peripheral feedback and central controls. The view proposed by Sherrington and reiterated by others (e.g. Jerge,
1964; Kawamura, 1967) that cyclic jaw movements and mastication have a
reflex basis must now be considered too simplistic and misleading. Central
factors, in addition to peripheral influences, are responsible for its genesis.

Peripheral and central control

In accord with findings related to swallowing, the experimental evidence (e.g.
Dellow and Lund, 1971) now indicates that the basic cyclical pattern of mastication is provided by a centrally programmed, neural pattern generator in
the reticular formation of the brain stem. The possibility that the generator
may be located within the v motor nucleus (Denavit-Saubié and Corvisier,
1972) was questioned, since it was felt that it had not been conclusively demonstrated in this study that the rhythmically discharging neurones recorded
were not, in fact, motoneurones and that the rhythm was related to mastication.

In contrast to swallowing, however, this central neural generator is sensitive
to, and in fact dependent on, sensory feedback for the genesis and continual
modification of the complex movement pattern. This has been pointed in
Goldberg's presentation (this volume), but his view that swallowing did not

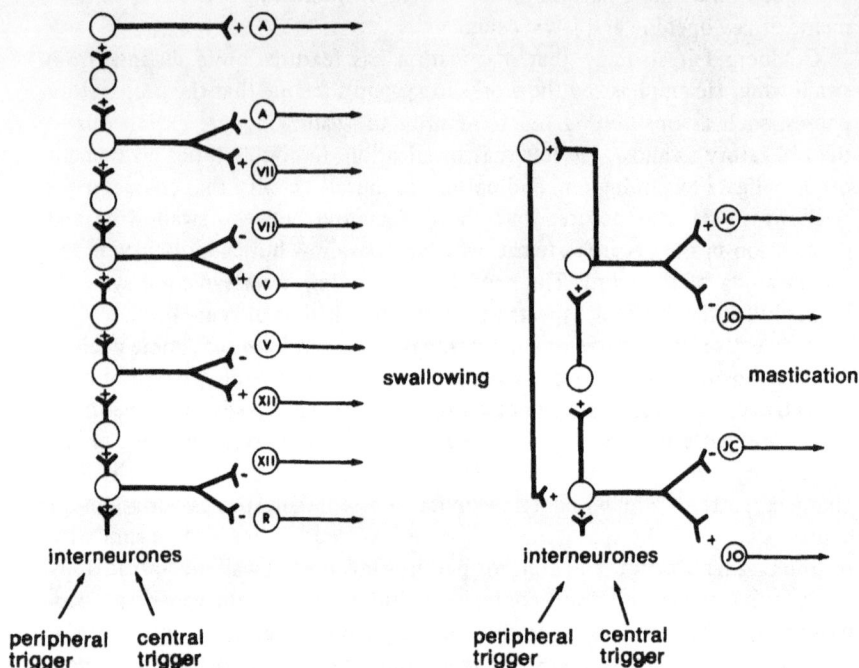

FIGURE 1 One possible scheme of central neural organization with characteristics that are similar for both swallowing and mastication. The motoneurones primarily involved are respiratory (R), hypoglossal (XII), trigeminal (V), facial (VII), ambiguus (A), jaw-opening (JO) and jaw-closing (JC). +: excitatory synapses; –: inhibitory synapses. The number of neurones in the internuncial chains by no means depicts actual numbers; numerous interneurones would be involved to provide the appropriate delays and sustained periods of excitation and inhibition. For ease of presentation, no central regulation of the lateral components of masticatory movements has been incorporated.

have an oscillating or alternating basis met with some criticism from Dubner, who felt that there was no evidence of the characteristics of the central patterning. Only the activity of the final motoneurone pools that are being influenced by the central generator(s) has received detailed study to date. Any difference between the central neural generators was inferred, he felt, and conceivably the pattern generators for mastication and swallowing are similar. A number of possibilities come to mind, and one of the more likely schemes is illustrated (Fig. 1).

In relation to a bulbar or higher centre for swallowing and mastication, Storey asked whether there may or may not be ontogenetic and/or phylogenetic differences. He mentioned respiration in cetaceans which apparently is

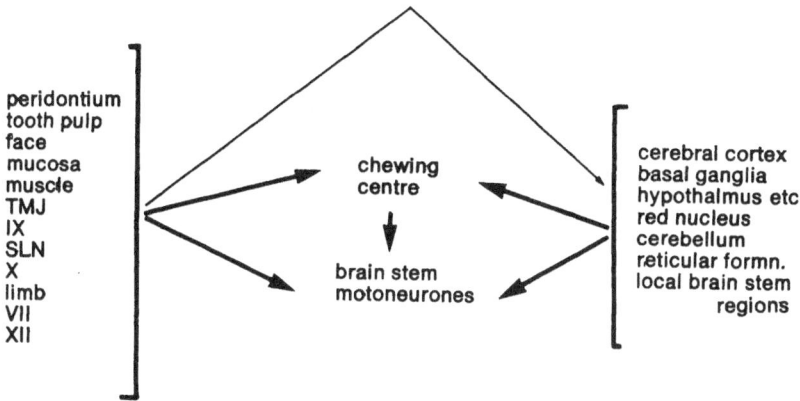

```
peridontium
tooth pulp
face
mucosa          →   chewing        ←        cerebral cortex
muscle              centre                   basal ganglia
TMJ                   ↓                      hypothalmus etc
IX                                           red nucleus
SLN                                          cerebellum
X               ←   brain stem     ←        reticular formn.
limb                motoneurones             local brain stem
VII                                              regions
XII
```

FIGURE 2 A number of peripheral sites are indicated that have been shown to exert a considerable and relatively direct influence over some or all of the motoneurone types involved in mastication. Many of these inputs can influence the activity of the chewing centre itself, or exert their effect by means of projections to one or more of the higher centres which have been shown to regulate the activity of the motoneurones relatively directly or via the chewing centre (for reference material, see Sessle and Kenny, 1973; Kawamura, 1974). As with Fig. 1, many more neurones than the ones indicated would be involved. IX: glossopharyngeal nerve; SLN: superior laryngeal nerve; X: vagus nerve; other abbreviations as in Fig. 1.

highly cortical and not organized at the brain stem level. Species differences in the ability to elicit masticatory movements were, in fact, cited (e.g. Kubota presentation, this volume), and Lund stressed that the movements elicited in some animals with cortical stimulation are natural and similar to masticatory movements. If the cortex is removed, and subcortical stimuli delivered, fractionation occurs, and the full pattern is no longer seen.

In addition to its likely action at the level of the pattern generator, sensory feedback might operate at least at two other levels (Fig. 2). First, it may influence higher centres such as cerebral cortex. In addition to the role of the cortex in the voluntary act of mastication, recent evidence (e.g. Lund and Lamarre, 1973; Lund and Sessle, 1974) indicates that the cortex may be receiving peripheral feedback from intraoral receptors during the masticatory act and be implicated in our ability to make contact with the food bolus and crush it. An obvious source of the information would be the periodontal receptors, providing a form of positive feedback on jaw-closing muscle activity. And at the level of the brain stem, periodontal receptors are capable of inducing powerful inhibitory effects on jaw-closing motoneurone activity. This then is an example of another level at which peripheral feedback might operate, and mastication may be over-ridden and interrupted, for example, by a noxious stimulus in the oral cavity.

Very little evidence is available of the extent to which learning is critical to the development and maintenance of mastication. Sessle and Dellow proposed that mastication in mammals might be considered to be fundamentally derived from suckling. Suckling is 'laid down' and apparently expressed very early in foetal life and would seem to provide a substrate of coordinated tongue, jaw, and facial muscle activity (see Humphrey, 1970; Dellow presentation, this volume). Upon such a suitable basis, factors such as maturation and changes in the oral environment (e.g. eruption of the teeth) might express themselves and so contribute to the total event which we know as mastication.

Note was made that eruption of the teeth constitutes a significant event in the development of the masticatory act. However, the fact that children with congenital absence of teeth can apparently chew would indicate that sensory feedback from the teeth is not all important. Nevertheless, children generally seem to be able to cope quite well with a new or changing dentition without developing mandibular dysfunction syndromes and bruxing problems seen in adults with permanent dentitions. Perhaps in infancy mastication is still being learned and thus is responsive to sensory feedback. However, because of the plasticity of the system, abnormal feedback patterns are not upsetting to most children. And 'bruxism' may be physiological rather than pathological, at least in children (see paper by Roydhouse, this volume).

Relative to learning in mastication, Storey pointed out that, whereas learning may occur very quickly in the young person when masticatory patterns are being formulated, it may occur rather slowly in the adult. This is one reason why he thought that in short-term anaesthetization studies of oral-facial tissues (e.g. Shaerer, Legault, and Zander, 1966) no changes occur in adult EMG patterns during mastication. It was felt that studies (e.g. deafferentation at various ages) aimed at determining the importance of oral-facial sensory feedback in the development of mastication are warranted in the chewing animal.

Considerable attention was also paid to the various types and sites of peripheral feedback, which were broadly divided into three categories: temporomandibular joint, muscle, and intraoral receptors. It was felt that the effects of natural stimulation of the joint receptors on reflex and masticatory activity had received too little attention (cf. Abe, Takata, and Kawamura, 1973) and only recently had any work been done of their influences on other muscles such as the tongue musculature (Lowe and Sessle, 1973).

The length or velocity information that derives from the muscle spindles in the elevator muscles has received some recent attention (e.g. Cody, Lee, and Taylor, 1972) although more definitive studies of these are needed with regard, for example, to identification, conduction velocity, and dynamic and static properties. Muscle tension receptors (Golgi tendon organs) also created comment in view of past uncertainty of their existence, and the apparent lack of effect on masseter motoneurones that might be attributed to them. However, further physiological studies are indicated in view of Lund's description earlier in the symposium of tendon organs in the jaw muscles.

There is no evidence of significant muscle afferent feedback from the depressor muscles, and only a very small number of muscle spindles have been found in them. These depressor muscles of the jaws are not nearly so large and powerful as their antagonists, the jaw-closing muscles. Apparently the large bulk and power of the elevators is counteracted by gravity and strong reflex excitatory influences from the periphery on the depressors, or at least the digastric. However, the peripheral, and central, influences on the lateral pterygoid have been sadly neglected in physiological studies. This lack of knowledge is partly due to limitations in recording, but in view of the importance of this muscle in lateral mandibular movements, it was felt imperative for studies to be carried out to define the neural mechanisms underlying its function.

Little evidence is also available of the reflex effects served by the group II, III, and IV muscle afferents (see Nakamura, Mori, and Nagashima, 1973). Much more study is also needed in this area in view of the neurophysiological and clinical significance of the nociceptive information carried by many of these afferents.

The role of intraoral receptors received considerable attention, and contrary to the view (mentioned above) of Schaerer et al. (1966), the general feeling was that disturbances seen in masticatory performance following trigeminal nerve anaesthetization are indications of the considerable influence that intraoral feedback exerts on mastication. Most of the discussion centred on feedback from periodontal receptors since their effects have received considerable attention from clinicians and neurophysiologists alike. The most powerful effect from the periodontium is inhibition of the jaw-closing muscles (see presentations by Goldberg; Greenwood and Sessle; Lund; this volume), but questions arose on a number of points related to this inhibition. Are different receptor types responsible for the different phases of inhibition? Can the early inhibitory phase produced in the jaw-closing muscles be overcome by positive feedback? This feedback might conceivably operate via the cortical level, for example, when crushing of food is desired. Does the late phase of inhibition provide a dampening which protects the masticatory apparatus from any excessive crushing force that may develop? And in cases of periodontal inflammation, are these effects exaggerated? We know little about the role played by nociceptors in the periodontium and their relationship in occlusal interferences to mastication and swallowing (the second workshop report gives further consideration to these aspects).

But just how critical is the periodontal input? It has been shown that other sites are also capable of initiating profound inhibitory effects. In the case of edentulous subjects, receptors in oral mucous membrane, temporomandibular joint and perhaps periosteum might be called upon to a greater extent to provide the sensory feedback necessary for mastication, protective reflexes, etc.

Just some of the questions that have considerable relevance to biological and clinical aspects of mastication have been mentioned above. By drawing attention to such unanswered problems in mastication, and also in swallowing, it is hoped that this workshop has served useful purposes, not only in providing a statement of our present level of knowledge of the programming and regulation of mastication and swallowing, but also in indicating valuable lines of future research in this area.

REFERENCES

Abe, K., Takata, M., and Kawamura, Y. 1973. A study on inhibition of masseter α-motor fibre discharges by mechanical stimulation of the temporomandibular joint in the cat. *Archs oral Biol.* 18: 301–4

Bradley, R.M., and Mistretta, C.M. 1973. Swallowing in fetal sheep. *Science* 179: 1016–17

Cody, F.W.J., Lee, R.W.H., and Taylor, A. 1972. A functional analysis of the components of the mesencephalic nucleus of the fifth nerve in the cat. *J. Physiol. (Lond.)* 226: 249–61

Dellow, P.G., and Lund, J.P. 1971. Evidence for central timing of rhythmical mastication. *J. Physiol. (Lond.)* 215: 1–13

Denavit-Saubié, M., and Corvisier, J. 1972. Cat trigeminal motor nucleus: rhythmic units firing in relation to opening movements of the mouth. *Brain Res.* 40: 500–3

Doty, .R.W. 1968. Neural organization of deglutition. In C.F. Code (ed.), *Handbook of Physiology.* Vol. IV, Sect. 6. Washington: Am. Physiol. Soc.

Doty, R.W., and Bosma, J.F. 1956. An electromyographics analysis of reflex deglutition. *J. Neurophysiol.* 19: 44–60

Doty, R.W., Richmond, W.H., and Storey, A.T. 1967. Effect of medullary lesions on coordination of deglutition. *Exp. Neurol.* 17: 91–106

Humphrey, T. 1970. Reflex activity in the oral and facial area of the human fetus. In J.F. Bosma (ed.), *Second Symposium on Oral Sensation and Perception.* Springfield, Ill.: Thomas

Jean, A. 1972. Localisation et activité des neurones deglutiteurs bulbaires. *J. Physiol. (Paris)* 64: 227–68

Jerge, C.R. 1964. The neurological mechanism underlying cyclic jaw movement. *J. prosth. Dent.* 64: 667–81

Kater, S.B., and Rowell, C.H.F. 1973. Integration of sensory and centrally programmed components in generation of cyclical feeding activity of Helisoma trivolvis. *J. Neurophysiol.* 36: 143–55

Kawamura, Y. 1967. Neurophysiological background of occlusion. *Periodont.* 5: 175–83

– 1974. Neurogenesis of mastication. In Y. Kawamura (ed.), *Frontiers of Oral Physiology.* Vol. 1. *Physiology of Mastication.* Basel: Karger

Kennedy, D., Calabrese, R.L., and Wine, J.J. 1974. Presynaptic inhibition: primary afferent depolarization in crayfish neurones. *Science* 186: 451–4

Lowe, A.A., and Sessle, B.J. 1973. Tongue activity during respiration, jaw opening, and swallowing in cat. *Canad. J. Physiol. Pharmacol.* 51: 1009–11

– 1974. Genioglossus activity during respiration, jaw opening and swallowing in cat and monkey. *J. dent. Res.* 53 (Special Issue): 201

Lund, J.P., and Lamarre, Y. 1973. The importance of positive feedback from periodontal pressoreceptors during voluntary isometric contraction of jaw closing muscles in man. *J. biol. bucc.* 1: 345–51

Lund, J.P., and Sessle, B.J. 1974. Oral-facial and jaw muscle afferent projections to neurones in cat frontal cortex. *Exp. Neurol.* 45: 314–31

Nakamura, Y., Mori, S., and Nagashima, H. 1973. Origin and central pathways of crossed inhibitory effects of afferents from the masseteric muscle on the masseteric motoneuron of the cat. *Brain Res.* 57: 29–42

Schaerer, P., Legault, J.V., and Zander, H.A. 1966. Mastication under anaesthesia. *Helv. odont. acta.* 10: 130–4

Sessle, B.J. 1973. Excitatory and inhibitory inputs to single neurones in the solitary tract nucleus and adjacent reticular formation. *Brain Res.* 53: 319–31

Sessle, B.J., and Kenny, D.J. 1973. Control of tongue and facial motility: neural mechanisms that may contribute to movements such as swallowing and sucking. In J.F. Bosma (ed.), *Fourth Symposium on Oral Sensation and Perception,* Bethesda: D.H.E.W.

Sessle, B.J., and Storey, A.T. 1972. Periodontal and facial influences on the laryngeal input to the brain stem of the cat. *Archs oral Biol.* 17: 1583–96

Sumi, T. 1971. Modification of cortically evoked rhythmic chewing and swallowing from mid-brain and pons. *Jap. J. Physiol.* 21: 489–506

– 1975. Coordination of neural organization of respiration and deglutition: its change with post-natal maturation. In J.F. Bosma and J. Showacre (eds.), *Development of Upper Respiratory Tract Form and Function: Implications for Sudden and Unexpected Infant Death,* in press

Yurkstas, A.A. 1965. The masticatory act. *J. prosth. Dent.* 15: 248–60

Is dental occlusal harmony obligatory for muscle harmony?

A.G. HANNAM

This report summarizes the response of the workshop group to the question, as well as the ensuing discussion of their observations by all the participants in the symposium. The original members of the workshop group were Drs R. Dubner, L.F. Greenwood, R.H. Roydhouse, N.R. Thomas, and A.G. Hannam (Chairman). What follows represents the Chairman's impression of the feelings expressed by the participants.

It soon became apparent that the question was not going to be answered satisfactorily, as current, factual information available in the area is inadequate. Nevertheless, the group did manage to come to grips with the question of what constitutes acceptable muscle function, and also with the role of measurement in the relationship between dental occlusion and the activity of the jaw musculature. In addition, a considerable effort was made to pinpoint principal areas of concern, and to suggest experimental approaches which might be used to eliminate them.

The participants began by attempting to define the terms 'neuromuscular balance' or 'muscle harmony,' using the data made available by electromyographic studies of the kind carried out by Møller (1966, 1974). Such data include observations of symmetry in function, timing, peak contraction values, duration of contraction, etc., and in many instances, the expected mean values for many of these variables. It was soon agreed that we needed a more flexible definition than one based upon stringent criteria such as these. Acceptable muscle function, it was decided, should be defined as any function that allows mastication and swallowing to occur in the absence of degenerative change in any other associated tissue. Now this is a very wide definition, but it does allow for marked differences in the patterns of muscle contraction between individuals, and even, for example, differences in sidedness in right-sided and left-sided chewing in the same individual.

The fact that the plasticity of the neuromuscular system allows it to adapt to morphological change very quickly and that the tissues adapt to altered muscle activity means that it may be a variable time before overt pathology becomes evident in either tissue. If the adaptation is successful, and non-progressive to the point of pathology, then one may consider the system to be in harmony, albeit altered. This means that measurement of all tissues becomes essential since periodic measures must be made in order to establish states and trends, and are therefore important in both human and animal situations alike. Since there are already, or should be, measures available for the states of certain tissues, for example the joint system and periodontal tissues, the degree of 'muscle harmony' can be assessed by measuring the neuromuscular system in function, and then comparing these measurements with those from other tissues. Radiography, tooth mobility, periodontal indices, presence and degree of pain are all examples of measures of the latter sort. If, as a result of periodic measurements of this kind, a monotonic trend is found in the behaviour of the neuromuscular system (either in jaw movement or muscle patterning) and an associated, deleterious, trend in the state of a related tissue or tissues is also discovered, then one can say that the system is not in a state of balance, and that the present situation is harmful to the patient. This approach does not point out causal relationships, of course, but it may give us some insight into the causal relationship between muscle function and dental occlusion.

The emphasis, then, was on the need for measuring the neuromuscular system in function, and one feeling of the group, which came out clearly, was the necessity for measuring parameters where possible under the most natural circumstances, whether the subjects be humans or experimental animals. The participants then started to consider the relationship between the teeth and neuromuscular system in normal function, and the experiments which they would like to see undertaken in the area. This was approached in a systematic fashion, and the studies of the effects of afferent inputs from the periodontal tissues and joints on normal neuromuscular function were considered first.

An initial point questioned the effect of periodontal denervation, for example, by extraction of the teeth. Other than the work of Black (1974), the group was not aware of any definitive studies to discover what happens functionally to a set of cells either in a sensory nucleus, or in cells further from that nucleus, for example efferent cells, when part of the afferent input is denervated. It was thought that it might be useful to carry out multiple dental extractions and then look not only for morphological changes, but also for functional changes in various brain stem nuclei. Such a procedure could alter motoneurone behaviour, or alternatively, have very little effect. Some felt that the change in function would not be significant. Others recalled a statement made earlier in the symposium by Møller, in which he reported histochemical changes in the muscles of edentulous patients (Ringquist, 1974). It

was reasoned that here there could be muscle changes simply because of altered demands placed upon muscles in denture-wearing patients, or because
the loss of periodontal afferents had altered motoneurone function in such a
way as to alter the muscle chemistry. There are of course problems such as
simultaneous destruction of pulpal afferents to be considered in studies along
these lines. The group, however, expressed a stronger interest in the answer to
the more general question, viz. what happens in the motoneurone pool as a
result of periodontal denervation, since it was felt that this had great significance with regard to the relationship between teeth and muscles.

Some of the techniques that have been used in experiments involving periodontal afferent neurones were then considered. Concern was expressed that
the results may depend very much upon the forms of stimulation used. The
usual stimuli have been taps and pushes to single teeth. Some studies have
been carried out on the effects of altered direction of stimulation at a single
unit level on first-order neurones, but there is very little information about
what happens to a population of neurones under these circumstances. Even
more important is the lack of work which has been done on lateral jaw reflexes in response to dental stimulation since these were first reported by
Lund, McLachlan, and Dellow (1971). The forms of stimulation used in the
past, and the amount of relevance these have to normal function, are therefore significant. What happens when multiple stimulation of teeth is employed, for example by tapping several teeth at the same time, or near-syn-
chronously, as often happens in mastication? Many researchers are familiar
with the upper canine tooth of the cat, which is a convenient tooth to stimulate from the point of view of access, but what sort of stimuli are being applied to this tooth, and how relevant is the entire masticatory system in the
carnivore to the complex system we know to exist in man? We have rarely
used posterior teeth in our studies. As a result there are strict limitations upon
how much we can extrapolate from the experiments carried out so far.

The discussion then moved to capsular afferents in the temporomandibular
joints, and concern was expressed about our understanding of the innervation
of the joints in the sense of the specification of their complete afferent innervation. Even assuming this has been defined for a given species (e.g. Shwaluk,
1971), just where do the different nerves go centrally? Do they all project to
the same area, or do they pass to different regions? If there are branches of
the masseter nerves and deep temporal nerves supplying the capsules, do they
go to the trigeminal (v) mesencephalic nucleus or to the v main sensory nucleus? If they go to the mesencephalic nucleus, is this how they reflexly influence the elevator jaw muscles? Degeneration studies are feasible in this area,
and should be carried out, preferably on both cat and primate. From the
physiological point of view, it was again felt that efforts should be made to

stimulate the joint receptors by more natural means. Most of the joint movements that occur during mastication are much smaller than many of those
used to elicit responses experimentally, and of course lateral jaw movements
must be recognized as normal for man, and impossible in the cat.

With regard to human studies involving the periodontal tissues and the
temporomandibular joints, the participants were impressed by the sort of approach presently being used by Lund with his tracking and perturbation experiments, and they felt that the use of similar experimental paradigms could be
profitable in the future, not only with the periodontal afferents, but also with
regard to joint afferents. For example, it should be fairly easy to employ displacement transducers instead of force transducers in experiments of an other-
wise basically similar design.

Without wishing to get too involved in a discussion of muscle studies *per se*,
since it was felt that these were more properly dealt with elsewhere, the group
nevertheless wished to stress some aspects of muscle contraction which it felt
to be intimately concerned with occlusion or occlusally related problems. In
particular, it was thought that the function of the lateral pterygoid has not
been precisely defined, especially with regard to its relationship to disc function and joint derangement, and the timing of events with respect to the head
of the condyle. Such studies are important, given the speculation and assumptions made in much of the literature concerned with aetiology of mandibular
dysfunction syndromes. Efforts should be made to reinforce and clarify our
present impression that there are two morphologically and functionally separate parts of the muscle (McNamara, 1973).

The medial pterygoid muscle was also thought to be poorly researched,
especially when one compares the information available about this muscle
with that collected for muscles such as the masseter and temporalis muscles.
This muscle has been associated with the mandibular dysfunction syndrome
by many people, and we thought that this should be looked at more carefully.
It should not be too difficult to do this in experimental animals, particularly
primates.

With regard to high-threshold afferents from muscle, it seems that a lot
more work is needed on defining what happens when these are activated,
since muscle pain is cited in the clinical literature as an important contributor
to dysfunction syndromes. At present we know very little about high-threshold afferent projections from muscle, brain stem reflexes associated with
these afferents, and the patterns of response in the elevator muscles of the
jaws.

Speculation has continued about potential experiments concerning the
central mechanisms involved in jaw movement and tooth contact. Following a
brief but spirited plea for some work to be carried out on the role of the cere-

bellum, the importance of finding out what happens to the system during sleep was discussed. A great deal happens in the neuromuscular system of the jaws during sleep, and this has a direct association, in many instances, with the occlusion of the teeth. It was considered that here it would be feasible to carry out experiments on both humans and animals. The few observations of human jaw muscle activity during sleep (e.g. Kraft, 1960) could be supplemented by additional study, and further animal experiments might perhaps be used to help answer the question of what happens to central and peripheral neurones and muscle function during the various sleep stages. Sessle cited studies (e.g. Chase and McGinty, 1970) indicating profound influences of sleep states on masseter and digastric reflex activity in animals.

The participants then began to suggest experiments which could be arranged to perturb the normal system in some way, for example by creating regional alterations or pathology and observing the effects. Here a variety of possibilities presented themselves. For example, there is a remarkable lack of definitive experiments designed to observe the effects of altered tooth surfaces and temporomandibular joint architecture on jaw muscle activity and jaw movement in normal function. These experiments are not difficult to perform, given adequate means of measuring the parameters involved, and they lend themselves very readily to the human subject. Technological advances are sufficient to allow such studies to be carried out at the present time, in that there are clearly established methods for recording both muscle and jaw responses in man (Møller, 1966; Gibbs et al., 1971; Gillings, Graham, and Duckmanton, 1973; Griffin and Malor, 1974). The questions one would like to see answered, then, are what specific changes in muscle function, and what specific changes in jaw movement patterns, are associated with specific alterations to the occlusion of the teeth, for example premature contacts, crossbites, non-working interferences, etc.? The use of longitudinal studies was also encouraged in this area, so that adaptive phenomena could be assessed. Most studies to date have not included enough simultaneously recorded parameters to permit multivariate analysis to be carried out on muscle, jaw movement and occlusal features of interest.

Matthews speculated whether there was any experimental evidence to substantiate the hypothesis that abnormalities of the occlusion can produce pathological changes in muscle or joint function. He pointed out that one of the problems in this area is the lack of estimation of occlusal disharmony in the dynamic sense, as opposed to the static measures which are generally used at present. Clinical experience tells us that teeth move when faulty restorations are placed in them, and although one may manipulate the jaw passively and demonstrate interferences as a result, these may not appear in normal function. Storey and Thomas quoted the work of Schaerer, Stallard, and

Zander (1967) as evidence that induced occlusal interferences could alter muscle patterns during mastication, and the group agreed that it would be informative to observe the effects of alterations such as these over prolonged periods. Ramfjord's work on bruxism (Ramfjord, 1961) was cited by Storey as a good example of muscle dysfunction related to occlusion of the teeth, in that both electromyographic changes in swallowing and patient comfort were significantly altered by selective grinding of a specific tooth, after more general attempts at equilibration.

On the subject of bruxism, no one appeared to be impressed with the thesis that the prime aetiological factor is dental malocclusion. Several in the group felt that, from the evidence available, both bruxing and clenching behaviour are very strongly related to suprasegmental mechanisms of the kind involved with stress, anxiety, and dreaming. Suggestions that minor occlusal discrepancies of the sort frequently mentioned in the clinical dental literature are responsible for bruxism are difficult to substantiate. Alteration or reduction of a bruxing habit by selective grinding of the teeth does not necessarily mean that malocclusion was the cause of the condition. It could simply mean that intraoral feedback has been drastically changed, and we know little about what effect drastic changes in afferent information *per se* have on habitual behaviour. The study of bruxism has also been confused by the different opinions held concerning its significance. Several participants were anxious to point out that it is very important to distinguish between bruxism, clenching, gnashing, and so on. A great deal of bruxism may be physiological in that children, primitive man, and other primates all show evidence of bruxing behaviour (e.g. see paper by Roydhouse, this volume).

Experiments involving noxious stimulation of the joint capsules in animals were then given some consideration. The close injection of kinins and other pain-producing substances into joint capsules, and the subsequent monitoring of the response in muscle groups around the joint, should provide some useful data.

There was a feeling in the group that the role of pain sensation in the temporomandibular joint itself may have been overemphasized. This idea is not new, in that muscles have been quoted as an alternative source of pain for quite a long time. In this regard, it would be useful to know whether, if one does get a specific change in one muscle, for example stiffness or soreness (caused, as it is often claimed, by occlusal imbalance of some sort), this change affects other muscles of the group. In other words, does pain in one muscle cause a specific distribution of change in other muscles? Bearing in mind experiments which have been carried out on muscles of the back and some of the head muscles, several participants suggested that systematic injection of pain-producing substances in specific muscles of the jaws and neck in man, and monitoring of the activity of several relevant muscles at the same time, would provide valuable information about the distribution of muscle effects in the localized spastic conditions frequently observed in mandibular dysfunction syndrome.

Storey speculated upon what one would consider as suitable evidence for muscle pathology, assuming that signs and symptoms such as tenderness, spasm, spasticity, or cramp would normally be considered adequate. He felt that there was a need to define what these are, since there can be derangements in the neurone, the neuromuscular junction, the muscle membrane and the actomyosin-ATP machinery, and that we should be more specific when we are talking about muscle pathology. With reference to muscle spasticity, Kawamura quoted Banasik and Laskin's work on long-term muscle stimulation in monkeys, and its association with resultant occlusal alterations (Banasik and Laskin, 1972). Storey further postulated that muscle splinting might be considered initially as physiological, a protective event, but that later, because of the hyperactivity, pain may result and produce pathological muscle spasm.

In an attempt to determine how one could determine whether certain kinds of obnoxious stimuli could openly result in changes producing pain and pathology, Dubner proposed two series of experiments, one in which the occlusion and joints would be manipulated to produce different alterations in muscle patterns during normal function, and another in which pathological changes would be induced in muscles and joints (e.g. by hypertonic saline injections) and the muscle patterns again observed. By comparing the results of these experiments, he suggested that one might be able to detect specific trends in occlusally related muscle patterns which could be considered pathological or potentially pathological.

The group then considered the effect of manipulating the central nervous system (by means of stress or anxiety) upon the muscles and upon the way the teeth make contact. Such experiments could be carried out in man by using artificial stress-inducing situations and monitoring jaw muscle activity by electromyography, clenching forces, or jaw movements. Indeed, some work of this kind is beginning to appear in the literature (e.g. Yemm, 1971). It was also felt that more use could be made of stressed primates, the 'executive' and orphan monkeys, in studies aimed at defining the role of tension and anxiety in parafunctional jaw movement and the extent that the teeth are involved in this relationship. With regard to the study of parafunctional jaw movements, it was suggested that more use could be made of pharmacological agents to induce various states of perturbation in the system, and that more study of jaw muscle activity related to aberrant sleep behaviour could prove useful.

The discussion concluded with the consideration of experiments designed to define the functional relationship between the v and cervical musculature, since some association between these muscle groups has been inferred in the literature on mandibular dysfunction syndromes, and has been discussed earlier in this symposium. It was noted that alterations may occur in the occlusion of the teeth following whiplash injury, and the speculation was made that these might occur either as a direct involvement of the mandibular suspensory apparatus during the traumatic episode, or as a result of muscle changes in the v system as a result of cervical nerve involvement. The point was made that patients suffering from this condition appear to restore their occlusion to normal, provided that treatment of the cervical syndrome is successful. However, there seems to be a sort of break-point at about three months post-injury. If the neck pain persists this long before it subsides, then the mandible seems to stay out of alignment. One might speculate that some form of central programming change has therefore been effected. Such cervical-v interactions, whether they initiate from the v area or from the cervical area, were viewed as being caused by three possible mechanisms.

The first possibility is one of referred pain, so that pain originating in one area would be interpreted as coming from the other and produce local postural changes in the latter region. The second possibility is that there are direct brain stem links between, for example, cervical neurones and v neurones. Although there is evidence of anatomical connections between the upper three cervical nerves and the v spinal nucleus, the functional significance of the connections is uncertain. In this regard, Sessle cited the recent unpublished observations by Abrahams and his colleagues at Queen's University, Kingston, which suggest that cervical neck muscle afferents project to the v spinal nucleus. Their interactions there, however, have yet to be studied. One of the problems to be faced is that, if there are functional connections between cervical afferents and v spinal neurones, then since most v spinal neurones appear to be inhibitory to the jaw elevator muscles, one would expect cervical afferent stimulation to have a similar effect; in fact, the opposite is seen in the clinic. Finally, the third possibility which could be interesting to explore experimentally was the proposal that nociceptive traffic from one area influences the motoneurones in the other area by a more diffuse circuitous route, that is the signals ascend suprasegmentally, and then descend again to reach the motoneurone pool concerned.

REFERENCES

Banasik, P.M., and Laskin, D.M. 1972. Production of masticatory muscle spasm and secondary tooth movement: an experimental model for MPD syndrome. *J. Oral Surg.* 30: 491–8

Black, R.G., 1974. A laboratory model for trigeminal neuralgia. In J. Bonica (ed.), *Advances in Neurology.* Vol. IV. *Pain.* New York: Raven Press

Chase, M.H., and McGinty, D.J. 1970. Somatomotor inhibition and excitation by forebrain stimulation during sleep and wakefulness: orbital cortex. *Brain Res.* 19: 127–36

Gibbs, C.H., Messerman, T., Reswick, J.B., and Derda, H.J. 1971. Functional movements of the mandible. *J. prosth. Dent.* 26: 604–20

Gillings, B.R.D., Graham, C.H., and Duckmanton, N.A. 1973. Jaw movements in young adult men during chewing. *J. prosth. Dent.* 29: 616–27

Griffin, C.J., and Malor, R. 1974. An analysis of mandibular movements. In Y. Kawamura (ed.), *Frontiers of Oral Physiology.* Vol. 1. *Physiology of Mastication.* Basel: Karger

Kraft, E. 1960. Uebereine Untersunchung der menschilchen Kaumuskeltätigkeit während des Nachtschlafes. *Stoma* 13: 7

Lund, J.P., McLachlan, R., and Dellow, P.G., 1971. A lateral jaw movement reflex. *Exp. Neurol.* 31: 189–99

McNamara, J.A., 1973. The independent functions of the two heads of the lateral pterygoid muscle. *Am. J. Anat.* 138: 197–206

Møller, E. 1966. The chewing apparatus. *Acta. physiol. scand.* 69: suppl. 280

— 1974. Action of the muscles of mastication. In Y. Kawamura (ed.), *Frontiers of Oral Physiology.* Vol. 1. *Physiology of Mastication.* Basel: Karger

Ramfjord, S.P. 1961. Bruxism, a clinical and electromyographic study. *J.A.D.A.* 62: 21–44

Ringquist, M. 1974. A histochemical study of temporal muscle fibres in denture wearers and subjects with natural dentition. *Scand. J. dent. Res.* 82: 28–39

Schaerer, P., Stallard, R.E., and Zander, H.A. 1967. Occlusal interferences and mastication: an electromyographic study. *J. prosth. Dent.* 17: 438–49

Shwaluk, S. 1971. Initiation of reflex activity from the temporomandibular joint of the cat. *J. dent. Res.* 50: 1642–6

Yemm, R. 1971. Comparison of the activity of left and right masseter muscles of normal individuals and patients with mandibular dysfunction during experimental stress. *J. dent. Res.* 50: 1320–3

What mechanisms contribute to the coordination of tongue movements during mastication and swallowing?

A.T. STOREY

The following report is a summary of the discussions initially given by Drs P. Dellow, S. Gobel, Y. Kawamura, A. Lowe, T. Sumi, and A. Storey (Chairman) on the above question and then in plenum session with all conference participants. We were asked to address ourselves to three questions: what do we know about the problem, what are some of the questions that need to be answered, and how do we go about answering them. Trends in research were identified but citations were not intended to be complete (see Kawamura, 1974, for some recent relevant review material).

The first consideration will be the anatomical substrate, which is Gobel's contribution. It should be pointed out that we all had a gut feeling that the primary coordination resided in the brain stem, and therefore both in our deliberation at the anatomical and at the physiological level we concentrated on the brain stem. The points Gobel made in his presentation were first that there is very little morphological data on the hypoglossal (xii) nucleus and the surrounding regions in the brain stem. There is less on the way in which these areas relate to each other on a structural basis, and there are no electron-micrograph studies of neuronal morphology and synaptic organization of first- and second-order afferents in the xii nucleus. The best material still goes back in many instances to Ramón y Cajal's work (1952). The xii nucleus itself is a homogeneous collection of large and small neurones. The large neurones are accepted as motoneurones. The question is not clear whether the small neurones are gamma motoneurones or whether they are interneurones. Speculation that these small neurones might be gamma motoneurones generated questions regarding the presence of spindles in the tongue. Kawamura pointed out the papers reporting muscle spindles in the tongues of humans and primates (Cooper, 1953; Bowman, 1968). One thing that characterizes the xii system as in all the other cranial motor nuclei is that there are no motoneurone axon collaterals, and so there is the question of how the inhibi-

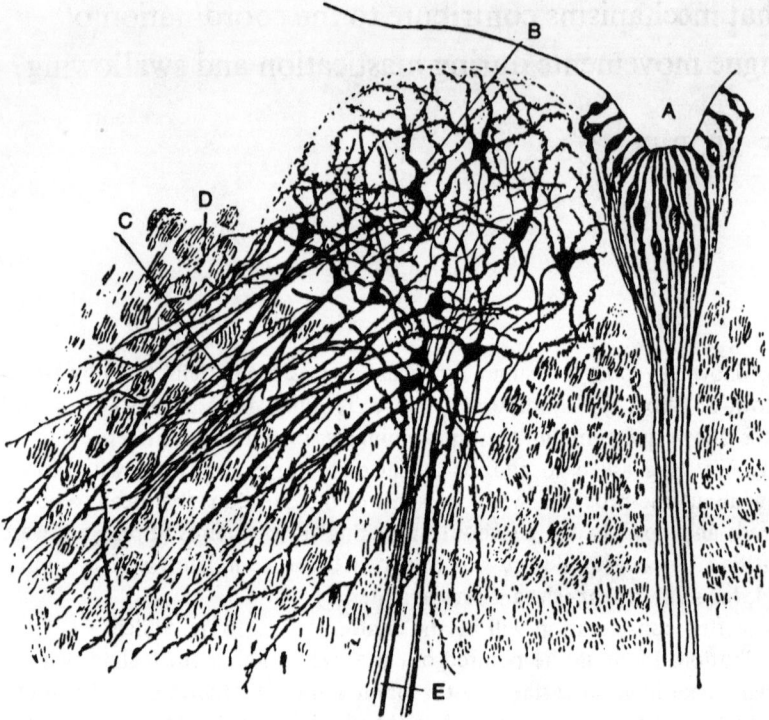

FIGURE 1   Section through the rostral third of the hypoglossal nucleus in an eight-day-old kitten. Golgi stain: A. median raphé with its epithelial extension; B. neurones of the hypoglossal nucleus; C. outer dendrites; D. central paths of the trigeminal, glossopharyngeal, and vagus nerves; E. hypoglossal root fibres. Reproduced from Rámon y Cajal, *Histologie du système neuveux de l'Homme et des Vertebrés*, Paris: Maloine Librairie. Courtesy of the author and the publisher.

tion which restricts the motor activity is brought about. One has to look elsewhere for that substrate. This is in contrast with ventral horn motoneurones.

One feature about the XII nucleus which comes across in a dramatic way is that the dendrites of many XII motoneurones sweep laterally towards the trigeminal (V) sensory nucleus and the solitary tract nucleus. These are well illustrated in a figure taken from Ramón y Cajal (1952). The dendrites (labelled C in Fig. 1) intersect the axons of second-order neurones whose cell bodies lie in the sensory nuclei of V and the solitary tract nucleus. These axons course through the reticular formation in bundles (D) and serve as one afferent input for the XII nucleus. Another possible input could be through reticular formation neurones located in the same region between the bundles. Gobel speculated that these reticular formation neurones may have dendrites going into the sensory nuclei but this has yet to be demonstrated. A third input may be the long axons descending into the xii nucleus from neurones in the v mesencephalic nucleus (tract of Probst). These axons course caudally through the brain stem and possibly send branches into the various motor nuclei. There is some evidence, from degeneration studies, that branches are given off these descending axons which may be heading for the xii nucleus. If this is so, such an input could be subserving a proprioceptive function. Sessle questioned a proprioceptive role for the tract of Probst on the basis of stimulation studies by Sumino and Nakamura (1973) of masseter nerve which demonstrated primarily inhibition of xii motoneurones and only at high thresholds. Gobel argued on the basis of earlier findings of a mesencephalic nucleus input into the supratrigeminal nucleus for a xii analogy.

Another point that Gobel made was that the xii nucleus itself is surrounded by a number of other nuclear masses. The suggestion has been made (e.g. Sumino and Nakamura, 1973) that the nucleus of Roller may act in a similar fashion to the supratrigeminal nucleus i.e. it may have an inhibitory role.

Recognizing the need for electronmicroscopic studies, Gobel tried to speculate upon what one might find. As a basis for this speculation he used electronmicroscopic studies which have been done on lumbar ventral horn cells and also his own work on the v nuclei. Primary afferent endings would be expected to have large endings containing large synaptic vesicles with multiple synaptic contacts on the basal dendritic trees of the motoneurones. Smaller axonal endings with small synaptic vesicles may form axoaxonal synapses on the afferent axons. Small endings with small synaptic vesicles could be expected on the soma and the more distal parts of the motoneurone dendritic tree.

Gobel then went on to identify what he considered the key problems in terms of the structural aspects of the coordination of tongue movements. The first one should be obvious – an electronmicroscopic study needs to be done, both of the xii nucleus and the surrounding nuclei. Second, it is obvious that one needs to test the various hypotheses regarding how the input gets into the xii neurones. Both structural as well as physiological studies will be needed. Finally, it will be necessary to study the morphology and axonal projections of the cell groups around the motor nucleus to try and determine their role in presumed inhibitory processes.

From the structural aspects we turned to the neurophysiological areas, to ascertain what was known, and what the problems were and how they might be attacked. This knowledge comes from three kinds of investigation: peripheral studies, brain stem studies, and higher centre effects. In the peripheral studies the input is based on either nerve stimulation or natural stimulation and the output on nerve recording, electromyogram (EMG), or observations of tongue movements. There is a great deal of data here, and only the general kinds of observations are summarized without citing who is responsible or identifying where there are differences between investigators.

Nerve stimulation may result in tongue protrusion or tongue retraction. Superior laryngeal nerve (SLN) stimulation tends to produce protrusion whereas lingual nerve and glossopharyngeal nerve (GPN) tend to produce retrusion. These effects can be conditioned from a number of areas by nerve stimulation. Lingual nerve, SLN, GPN, masseteric nerve, upper lip, and tooth pulp stimulation results in an initial facilitation and then a long-lasting inhibition of up to 400 msec; infraorbital nerve and tooth tap stimulation result in an initial facilitation and short-lasting inhibition of either tongue protrusion or retrusion (see Schmitt, Yu, and Sessle, 1973).

Stimulation of the lingual nerve and GPN will produce EMG changes. These may be conditioned by digastric nerve or masseteric nerve stimulation, resulting in inhibition of the EMG. However, the specific muscle and the nature of the resulting movement frequently have not been specified in these studies. Finally, XII nerve stimulation itself will produce reflex activity in the styloglossus muscle, but high-intensity stimulation is required, and there is some variability in findings of investigators.

There are problems in the interpretation of these findings which explains why they have not been detailed further. One is that the nerves stimulated are mixed nerves. The number and population of fibres stimulated are uncertain. There is no way of knowing, from the effects, whether these effects seen in the tongue are a protective reflex, or whether they represent a pathway which might be utilized in mastication or swallowing.

When one turns to natural stimulation, there are EMG findings that genioglossus shows rhythmic activity with respiration (Lowe and Sessle, 1973). Lund reported he had observed the same response in the XII nerve and suggested that it occurs under conditions when auxiliary muscles are recruited to increase ventilation. Lowe indicated that the response is most marked in the posterior part of the tongue. The genioglossus EMG is also sensitive to change in position of the jaw. Lowe reported that this proprioceptive input arises from the temporomandibular joint.

Turning to the numerous brain stem studies, one finds, as expected, effects to both nerve stimulation and natural stimulation. Whole nerve stimulation of the lingual nerve, masseteric nerve, GPN, SLN, the vagus and XII nerve itself will produce facilitatory and/or inhibitory effects depending in part on the nerve stimulated and also the investigator. Most investigators have not indicated whether they were recording from protrusive or retrusive motoneurones, so the functional significance of these various effects cannot be fully specified from their studies. There are obviously inputs also from the respiratory centre, swallowing centre, and the masticatory centre, but any information on these is scarce. There are problems in these studies as before, viz. with whole nerve stimulation, what is being stimulated, and what does it mean?

Sumi reported that in his recordings from XII motoneurones he occasionally observed a response that he thought was reminiscent of a Renshaw cell. In these experiments the XII nerve was stimulated and intracellular recordings made from neurones in the nucleus. In nine cells a repetitive train of spikes occurred on the crest of the EPSP with latencies of less than 1 msec to 6 msec (Sumi, 1969) to a single stimulus. The location of such cells within the XII nucleus has not been established.

The XII neurones have also been examined with natural stimulation. Tactile stimulation of the tongue has been shown to produce activity in XII motoneurones, and Kawamura reported that gustatory stimulation of the tongue will produce activity in the XII nerve. There is good electrophysiological evidence that there are no direct monosynaptic connections from the lingual or masseter nerve to XII motoneurones. This implies that there are no spindle afferent inputs onto XII motoneurones. Gobel wondered if this depended on the species studied and Lund questioned whether a small number of spindle afferents, which might miss detection, would have a significant effect anyway on the XII motoneurone pool.

There has not been much study of higher centre effects, although several workers have shown XII neurone activity locked to mastication and swallowing. Morimoto and Kawamura (1973) have demonstrated tongue protrusion and retraction and lapping on orbital gyrus stimulation, and Porter (1967) has recorded short-latency intracellular hypoglossal IPSPs on cortical stimulation. There are apparently no studies of the results of stimulating other higher centres, e.g. subcortical regions, cerebellum, etc. A great need was felt to refine some of the stimulating and recording techniques, with inputs better restricted, and motor nerves and lingual muscles specifically identified.

There is not much work to discuss with regard to human studies in this area. Such studies also suffer from the difficulty of controlling the circumstances under which data are collected, and in their interpretation. There have been EMG studies of tongue muscles in man (Bole and Lessler, 1966; Cunningham and Basmajian, 1969), and Cleall's group in Manitoba has used a cineradiographic approach. With respect to this latter technique, Matthews asked how useful it was in providing information in the diagnosis and treatment of tongue problems, e.g. tongue thrusting, when committees asked to assess experiments on humans are concerned about radiation. Storey felt the radiation risk had been reduced with image intensification, but that only seeing structures in two dimensions limits its usefulness in studying the tongue. Lowe argued that the technique has little clinical usefulness in assessing tongue problems, particularly if the head is oriented using ear rods or if radiopaque materials of unusual consistency are used.

Sessle reported that the first workshop group had discussed the quasi-obligate pattern of swallowing, and brought up the question of whether the genioglossus was an obligatory muscle in swallowing. Storey indicated that it would depend on whether the muscle was participating prior to or in the buccopharyngeal stage of swallowing. It might participate in an elective fashion before a certain time and thereafter as an obligate muscle of the swallow. Lowe reported that in the cat and monkey there are two types of genioglossus activity – activity that might precede the tightly programmed swallow and activity that was part of it. They seemed to be two different things. Although the situation in man is not known, it could account for success with myofunctional therapy in some cases and failure in others. However, Lowe pointed out that it is uncertain whether tongue-thrusting causes orthodontic problems in the first place. The posture of the tongue and lips may be more important.

To a question from Matthews asking whether attempts had been made to train animals to modify their basic swallowing pattern, Lowe replied that he did not think so. Storey thought such an investigation would be more meaningful if one were able to develop a tongue-thrusting animal. Lund suggested a spout with a ball-bearing which would have to be pressed in order to obtain water. Lowe was concerned about the jaw opening altering tongue position in this training situation, and Roydhouse pointed out that this would only be training tongue activity preliminary to the swallow. Goldberg asked whether neurologists see any modifications in swallowing patterns, particularly with respect to the role of the tongue. He was thinking of problems in swallowing which might occur in children with cerebral palsy, or poliomyelitis. Kenny (unpublished observations) has found that swallowing is usually normal in lateral-facial dysplasia, but abnormal swallowing may be seen in children following cerebro-vascular accidents. Tongue function appears to be affected when there is damage to XII motoneurones or cerebellum as a result of cerebral anoxia or kernicturus at birth or trauma later in life.

Sessle identified the contrasting roles of feedback in swallowing compared to mastication. Sensory feedback is available from V, GPN, SLN afferents, etc. Mastication has a central component upon which is imposed sensory feedback. People normally do not bite their tongues while chewing but do so if the lingual nerves are anaesthetized. In contrast central programming would appear to dominate for tongue coordination during swallowing with little importance attached to sensory feedback. Dubner emphasized again the importance of defining which tongue movements are part of the buccopharyngeal stage.

Relative to the problems in this area, the cause of tongue-thrusting was brought up. In an attempt to answer this question, some thought that an attempt should be made to find out from what part of the central nervous system the signals come that activate the genioglossal neurones responsible for the protraction. Are they coming from receptors in and around the mouth, from the swallowing centre itself, or from higher centres? It was agreed that it would be necessary to document better human tongue activity, concentrating on specific muscles. It would be valuable to be able to view the tongue directly without disrupting its activity, and the possibility of using fibre optics was raised, for example, by a nasal approach. Ideally, one needs a non-invasive three-dimensional monitor to look at tongue activity. It would also be helpful to look at the effect of changes in tactile input and changes in vertical dimension on this clinical problem.

On the question of lingual receptors and their role in tongue coordination, we were aware of the arguments relative to proprioreceptors in the tongue versus tactile receptors on the tongue as being responsible for feedback. The question of lingual proprioception is still open. Kawamura and Morimoto (1973) have reported that there are some afferent fibres in the lingual, glossopharyngeal and hypoglossal nerves which respond to forward stretch of the tongue.

Finally, with regard to the interplay between mastication, swallowing, and respiration, Sumi provided some evidence of interaction (Fig. 2). Figure 2 shows masticatory movements elicited by cortical stimulation in a lightly anaesthetized rabbit. Water was injected in increasing amounts into the oropharynx during this activity. A small volume of water does not disrupt mastication very much, whereas a large volume disrupts it considerably. This would indicate that mastication and swallowing are interacting. The question that might be asked is 'what about respiration?' Is this being interrupted at the same time? Is there interaction between mastication, swallowing, and respiration?

Dellow wanted to emphasize the need to look at the tongue in relation to respiratory activity - for example, the effects of gas tension and also laryngeal airway maintenance, upper airway resistance, etc. This has obvious implications for sudden unexplained deaths in infants and also may provide some insight into how tongue posture fails in the Pierre-Robin syndrome. It is also felt necessary to look at synergies engaging the tongue other than mastication, swallowing, and respiration, and Kawamura felt strongly about this. Much of what we have been talking about may not necessarily be part of mastication or swallowing, but may have more to do with gagging or vomiting or speaking.

Three other major problem areas were identified. Phylogenetic studies should be undertaken since the tongue varies greatly in size, shape, movement,

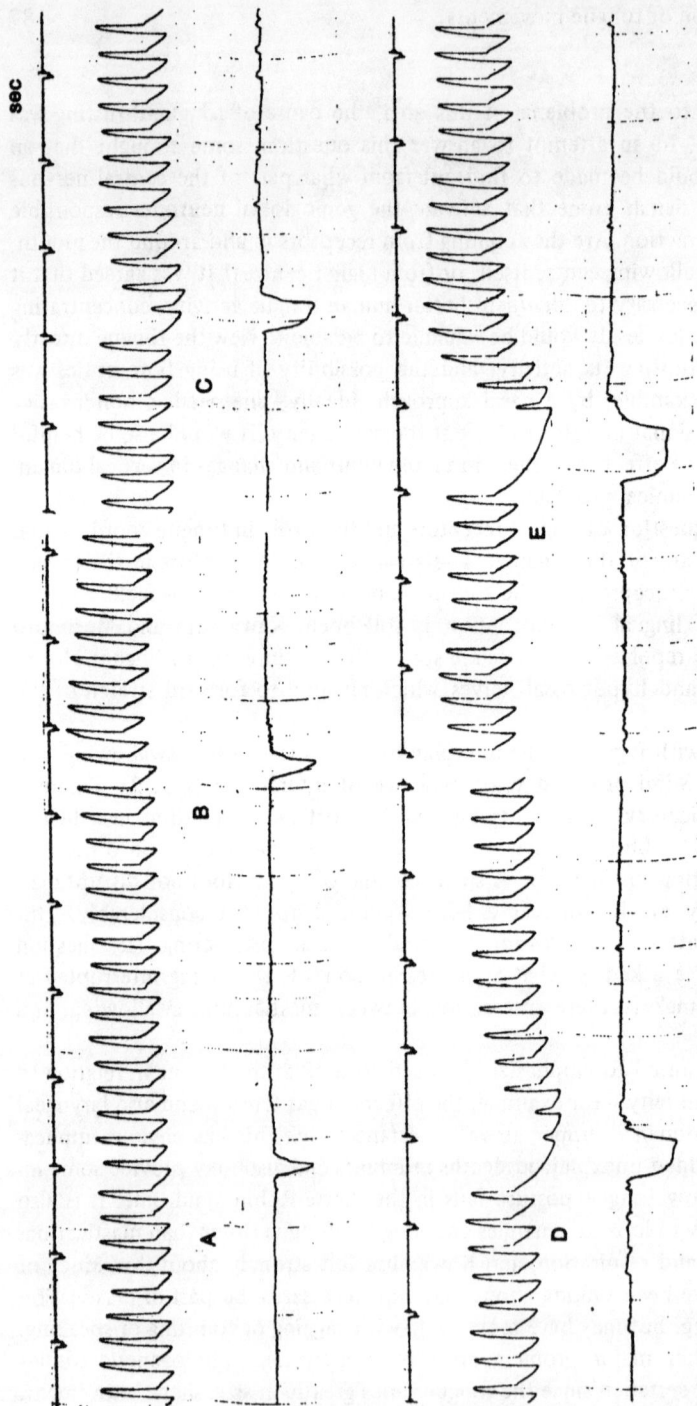

FIGURE 2 Upper trace: rhythmic jaw movements (mastication) induced by cortical stimulation with tetanic electrical pulses (duration: 0.2 msec; frequency: 50 Hz). Jaw closing, upward. Lower trace: swallowing induced by cortical stimulation alone at 'A' or induced by squirting water (amount was increased from 'B' to 'E') into the oropharynx. Rostral movement of the thyroid cartilage, downward. (Sumi, T., unpublished data from rabbit).

and function in different animals. Ontogenetic studies would be useful, with regard to the development of the nervous system, at both light and electron-microscopic levels. Finally, there was a suggestion that we should look at different muscle types, perhaps fast and slow muscles in the tongue, and examine the differences in the mix at various ages and with different functional tongue derangements.

REFERENCES

Bole, C.T., and Lessler, M.A. 1966. Electromyography of the genioglossus muscles in man. *J. Appl. Physiol.* 21: 1695-8

Bowman, J.P. 1968. Muscle spindles in the intrinsic and extrinsic muscles of the rhesus monkey's (macaca mulatta) tongue. *Anat. Rec.* 161: 483-8

Cooper, S. 1953. Muscle spindles in the intrinsic muscles of the human tongue. *J. Physiol. (Lond.)* 122: 193-202

Cunningham, D.P., and Basmajian, J.V. 1969. Electromyography of genioglossus and geniohyoid muscles during deglutition. *Anat. Rec.* 165: 401-10

Kawamura, Y. 1974. Neurogenesis of mastication. In Y. Kawamura (ed.), *Frontiers of Oral Physiology.* Vol. 1. *Physiology of Mastication.* Basel: Karger

Kawamura, Y., and Morimoto, T. 1973. Neurophysiological mechanisms related to reflex control of tongue movements. In J.F. Bosma (ed.), *Fourth Symposium on Oral Sensation and Perception.* Bethesda: D.H.E.W.

Lowe, A.A., and Sessle, B.J. 1973. Tongue activity during respiration, jaw opening and swallowing in the cat. *Canad. J. Physiol. Pharmacol.* 51: 1009-11

Morimoto, T., and Kawamura, Y. 1973. Properties of tongue and jaw movements elicited by stimulation of the orbital gyrus in cat. *Archs oral Biol.* 18: 361-72

Porter, R. 1967. Cortical actions on hypoglossal motoneurons in cats: a proposed role for a common internuncial cell. *J. Physiol. (Lond.)* 193: 295-308

Ramón y Cajal, S. 1952. *Histologie du Système Nerveux de l'Homme et des Vertébrés.* Madrid: Instituto Ramón y Cajal

Schmitt, A., Yu, S.-K.J., and Sessle, B.J. 1973. Excitatory and inhibitory influences from laryngeal and orofacial areas on tongue position in the cat. *Archs oral Biol.* 18: 1121-30

Sumi, T. 1969. Functional differentiation of hypoglossal neurons in cats. *Jap. J. Physiol.* 19: 55-67

Sumino, R., and Nakamura, Y. 1973. Synaptic potentials of hypoglossal
    motoneurons and a common inhibitory interneuron in the trigemino-
    hypoglossal reflex. *Brain Res.* 73: 439–54

Index